Evidence-based Care for Breastfeeding Mothers

A resource for midwives and allied healthcare professionals

Maria Pollard

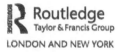

Routledge
Taylor & Francis Group

LONDON AND NEW YORK

First published 2012
by Routledge
2 Park Square, Milton Park, Abingdon, Oxon OX14 4RN

Simultaneously published in the USA and Canada
by Routledge
711 Third Avenue, New York, NY 10017

Routledge is an imprint of the Taylor & Francis Group, an informa business

British Library Cataloguing in Publication Data
A catalogue record for this book is available from the British Library

Library of Congress Cataloging in Publication Data
Pollard, Maria, 1965–
    Evidence-based care for breastfeeding mothers: a resource for midwives
    and allied healthcare professionals / Maria Pollard.
    p. cm.
    Includes bibliographical references.
    1. Breastfeeding promotion. 2. Breastfeeding – Health aspects.
    3. Evidence-based medicine. 4. Allied health personnel. 5. Midwifery.
    I. Title.
    [DNLM: 1. Breast Feeding. 2. Allied Health Personnel. 3. Lactation.
    4. Maternal Health Services. 5. Midwifery. WS 125]
    RJ216.P65 2011
    649′.33–dc22   2010053478

ISBN13: 978-0-415-49906-4 (hbk)
ISBN13: 978-0-415-49907-1 (pbk)
ISBN13: 978-0-203-80893-1 (ebk)

Typeset in Garamond
by Florence Production Ltd, Stoodleigh, Devon

Contents

Illustrations

Boxes

Preface

Healthcare professionals' lack of knowledge and skills to support mothers to breastfeed their infants has been identified as a major contributing factor to low rates of initiation and duration of breastfeeding, leading to inconsistent and inaccurate advice (Sikorski *et al.*, 2002; Hall-Moran *et al.*, 2004; Renfrew *et al.*, 2005). This is a key public health problem for society and therefore has major implications for service providers, as well as universities, in relation to how students are taught about breastfeeding within the pre-registration curriculum and how midwives, health visitors and other healthcare professionals keep themselves up to date.

Battersby (2002) suggested that midwives are exposed to similar experiences of breastfeeding, and cultural influences, as the mothers they care for, which may therefore affect professional practice in both positive and negative ways. There have been a number of studies carried out to identify the reasons for midwives' lack of knowledge and skill, most of which culminates in recommendations being made to improve post-registration education related to breastfeeding (Cantrill *et al.*, 2003; Renfrew *et al.*, 2005; McFadden *et al.*, 2007). However, it was not until the introduction of the UNICEF UK Baby Friendly Initiative (BFI) *Best Practice Standards into Breastfeeding Education for Student Midwives and Health Visitors* (UNICEF, 2002; updated 2008), and more recently the Nursing and Midwifery Council (NMC) *Essential Skills Clusters Circular* (NMC, 2007), that the focus has moved to pre-registration education.

There is a dearth of information available on how breastfeeding is specifically taught in midwifery curricula in the United Kingdom (UK) today, which may reflect the lack of value placed on breastfeeding by society (Dykes, 2003). However, the evidence that is available relating to breastfeeding education in the UK focuses on the lack of formal education opportunities and 'chaotic' learning environments (Renfrew *et al.*, 2005; Smale *et al.*, 2006; Jackson, 2007; McFadden *et al.*, 2007).

These findings were similar to multidisciplinary studies in other countries with poor breastfeeding rates, which found that health professionals felt they did not have sufficient education and training to support women (Freed *et al.*, 1995; Cantrill *et al.*, 2003; Al-Nassaj *et al.*, 2004). Freed *et al.* (1996) conducted a study of five American nursing programmes and reported that, although most students attended lectures on breastfeeding, only a quarter gained instruction through clinical activity. This is supported by Hellings and Howe (2004), who found that participants felt their personal experiences of breastfeeding to be the most valuable source of information; however, they did not have the ability to answer questions on breastfeeding management correctly.

Renfrew *et al.* recommend that:

> universities should be fundamental in providing opportunity for pre and post registration education for all health professionals, perhaps adopting the *UNICEF UK Baby Friendly Standards for Pre-registration Education* (UNICEF, 2002) as a framework, and developing self-study approaches and close links with clinical areas to enable supervised practice.
>
> (2005, p. 87)

The content of this book reflects the UNICEF UK BFI *Best Practice Standards for Higher Education Institutions* (2008) and will address the following 18 outcomes to ensure that students, midwives and other related healthcare professionals are equipped with essential knowledge and skills to enable them to support breastfeeding mothers through the application of evidence-based knowledge to clinical situations.

1 Understand the importance of breastfeeding and the consequences of not breastfeeding in terms of health outcomes.
2 Have developed an in-depth knowledge of the physiology of lactation and be able to apply this in practical situations.
3 Be able to recognise effective positioning, attachment and suckling and to empower mothers to develop the skills necessary for them to achieve these for themselves.
4 Be able to demonstrate knowledge of the principles of hand expression and have the ability to teach these to mothers.
5 Understand the potential impact of delivery room practices on the well-being of mother and baby and on the establishment of breastfeeding in particular.
6 Understand why it is important for mothers to keep their babies near them.
7 Understand the principle of demand feeding and be able to explain its importance in relation to the establishment and maintenance of lactation.

8 Be equipped to provide parents with accurate, evidence-based information about activities which may have an impact on breastfeeding.

9 Understand the importance of exclusive breastfeeding for the first six months of life and possess the knowledge and skills to enable mothers to achieve this.

10 Understand the importance of timely introduction of complementary foods and of continuing breastfeeding during the weaning period, into the second year of life and beyond.

11 Understand the importance of community support for breastfeeding and demonstrate an awareness of the role of community-based support networks, both in supporting women to breastfeed and as a resource for health professionals.

12 Be able to support mothers who are separated from their babies (e.g. on admission to SCBU [special care baby unit], when returning to work) to initiate and/or maintain their lactation and to feed their babies optimally.

13 Be able to demonstrate a knowledge of alternative methods of infant feeding and care which may be used where breastfeeding is not possible and which will enhance the likelihood of a later transition to breastfeeding.

14 Identify babies who require a managed approach to feeding and describe appropriate care.

15 Know about the common complications of breastfeeding, how these arise and how women may be helped to overcome them.

16 Understand the limited number of situations in which exclusive breast-feeding is not possible and be able to support mothers in partial breastfeed-ing or artificial feeding in these circumstances.

17 Appreciate the main differences between the WHO *International Code of Marketing of Breast-milk Substitutes* and the relevant current UK legislation and understand the relevance of the Code to their own work situation.

18 Be thoroughly conversant with the BFI best practice standards, understand the rationale behind them and what the BFI seeks to achieve through them and be equipped to implement them in their own workplace, with appropriate support from colleagues.

(Appendix 1 provides a breakdown and further explanation of the components of each outcome.)

The book will begin by putting breastfeeding into its socio-political context, and then will set out the essential knowledge and skills required to promote, initiate and support breastfeeding mothers in the early days. This will lead on to the management of common problems and supporting breastfeeding mothers and babies with special needs, which will include alternative methods of infant feeding when breastfeeding is not possible. The book will then move on to look at the older baby in relation to when and how to commence weaning and ongoing support of mothers in the community. The book concludes with a chapter on developing knowledge and skills to support breastfeeding mothers.

Each chapter will be mapped to the appropriate UNICEF BFI (2008b) learning outcomes and the main text will be evidence-based, relating the theory to clinical practice. However, it is evident that in many areas of breast-feeding management there is a dearth of evidence. Each chapter includes key fact boxes, clinical activities, diagrams and photographs where appropriate. Each chapter will be consolidated with a quiz, scenarios or reflective questions, and answers to these will be found at the end of the book. Useful resources will also be listed at the end of each chapter with a complete reference list and a glossary at the end of the book.

Acknowledgements

I would like to thank the following for giving permission to reproduce material: Medela, Karen McKay NHS Highland, TIPS, and special thanks to the UNICEF UK Baby Friendly Initiative.

Sincere thanks to my midwifery colleagues at the University of the West of Scotland for their support and advice.

A special thank you to Tony for his support and patience.

Abbreviations

ABM	Association of Breastfeeding Mothers
AED	anti-epileptic drug
APGAR	appearance, pulse, grimace, activity, respiration (from Apgar, its inventor)
ARV	antiretroviral
BALT	bronchus-associated lymphatic tissue
BFI	Baby Friendly Initiative
BFLG	Baby Feeding Law Group
BFM	*Breastfeeding Manifesto*
BFN	Breastfeeding Network
BMA	Baby Milk Action
BMI	body mass index
BPA	bisphenol-A
DH	Department of Health
ESC	Esssential Skills Cluster
FIL	feedback inhibitor of lactation
FSA	Food Standards Agency
FSID	Foundation for the Study of Infant Deaths
GALT	gut-associated lymphatic tissue
GP	general practitioner
HBIG	hepatitis B immune globulin
HCV	hepatitis C virus
HE	higher education
HEAT	health improvement, efficiency, access, treatment
HPL	human placental lactogen
HSE	Health and Safety Executive
IBFAN	International Baby Food Action Network
IFAS	Infant Feeding Attitude Scale
LAM	lactational amenorrhoea method
NAS	neonatal abstinence syndrome

NCT	National Childbirth Trust
NICE	National Institute for Health and Clinical Excellence
NMC	Nursing and Midwifery Council
PCOS	polycystic ovary syndrome
PIF	prolactin-inhibiting factor
RCM	Royal College of Midwifery
SACN	Scientific Advisory Committee on Nutrition
SCBU	special care baby unit
SIDS	sudden infant death syndrome
sIgA	secretory immunoglobin A
SIGN	Scottish Intercollegiate Guidelines Network
TAMBA	Twins and Multiple Births Association
TB	tuberculosis
UK	United Kingdom
UKAMB	United Kingdom Association for Milk Banking
UNICEF	United Nations Children's Fund
WABA	World Alliance for Breastfeeding Action
WHA	World Health Assembly
WHO	World Health Organization

Chapter 1 Putting breastfeeding into context

- Learning outcomes
- The benefits of breastfeeding
- Economic and environmental factors
- Who breastfeeds?
- UNICEF UK Baby Friendly Initiative
- Global and national strategies
- Concluding comments
- Practice questions
- Resources

Breastfeeding cannot be considered as a standalone subject when culture, social support and healthcare professionals' knowledge and skills clearly have such a great impact on initiation and duration of breastfeeding rates in the UK (Renfrew *et al.*, 2005). Breastfeeding must be placed in the wider socio-political context to understand why mothers make the choices they do with regard to infant feeding and to enable healthcare professionals to adequately support them in practice. The aim of this chapter is to identify the role breastfeeding has in promoting public health and reducing health inequalities for both mother and infant by exploring the health benefits of breastfeeding and the dangers of not doing so. It goes on to explore the results of the *Infant Feeding Survey 2005* (Bolling *et al.*, 2007) to highlight which mothers are most likely to breastfeed, and those least likely initiate breastfeeding, or who do so for a shorter period of time. This information is useful for both strategic developments of services as well as for planning individualised care. This chapter also introduces some of the main global, national and local strategies to promote, support and protect breastfeeding.

Learning outcomes

By the end of this chapter you will be able to:

* identify the health benefits of breastfeeding for mother and infant;
* recognise the socio-economic characteristics of mothers who choose whether to breastfeed or not;
* describe the BFI best practice standards for healthcare facilities and education;
* discuss the importance of global, national and local policies and guidelines to encourage and support breastfeeding.

The benefits of breastfeeding

The World Health Organization (WHO, 2002) recommends exclusive breast-feeding for the first six months of life and to continue for two years and beyond, because breastmilk is perfectly balanced to meet the nutritional needs of the newborn and is the only food required until six months of age. Breastmilk has the advantage of being readily available, at no cost, and delivered on demand and at the right temperature, and the infant is able to regulate the amount required at each feed. The properties of breastmilk are exclusive, cannot be replicated by formula milk (see Chapter 2) and confer many benefits on both

---

Mapping the UNICEF UK BFI educational outcomes

1 Understand the importance of breastfeeding and the consequences of not breastfeeding in terms of health outcomes.

8 Be equipped to provide parents with accurate, evidence-based information about activities which may have an impact on breastfeeding.

9 Understand the importance of exclusive breastfeeding for the first six months of life and possess the knowledge and skills to enable mothers to achieve this.

17 Appreciate the main differences between the WHO *International Code of Marketing of Breast-milk Substitutes* and the relevant current UK legislation and understand the relevance of the Code to their own work situation.

18 Be thoroughly conversant with the BFI best practice standards, understand the rationale behind them and what the BFI seeks to achieve through them and be equipped to implement them in their own workplace, with appropriate support from colleagues.

mother and infant. Despite this, the WHO (2010a) estimates that only 40 per cent of infants worldwide are exclusively breastfed for six months.

In 2007, Ip *et al.* conducted a systematic review of the evidence on the effects of breastfeeding on short- and long-term infant and maternal health in developed countries. For the infant, they suggested that breastfeeding reduces the risk of:

- diarrhoea and chest infections;
- atopic dermatitis and asthma;
- obesity and type I and II diabetes;
- childhood leukaemia;
- sudden infant death syndrome (SIDS);
- necrotising enterocolitis.

The UK is facing an obesity epidemic that is predicted to increase to one in three adults by 2012. Obesity is associated with an increased risk of hypertension, type II diabetes, heart disease and some cancers. Numerous studies have found that prolonged or 'dose-related' breastfeeding reduces the risk of obesity and that breastfed children are leaner than those who were never breastfed (Armstrong and Reilly, 2002). The *Millennium Cohort Study* (Sherburne-Hawkins *et al.*, 2008) found that 23 per cent of children in the UK under the age of three years were overweight, 5 per cent of whom were classed as obese. They highlighted contributing factors as not breastfeeding, breastfeeding for four months or less and introducing solid foods before four months of age. These findings support the results from a study of four-year-old children from low-income families in the United States by Grummer-Strawn and Mei (2004), which concluded that prolonged breastfeeding was associated with a reduced risk of being overweight.

Leon-Cava *et al.* (2002) and Kramer *et al.* (2008) suggest a link between intellectual and motor development and dose-related breastfeeding. It is thought this could be due to the long-chain polyunsaturated fatty acids in breastmilk as well as the psychosocial stimulation and bonding conferred by breastfeeding.

Breastfeeding also confers benefits on the mother by regulating fertility (WHO, 2010a) and reducing the risk of osteoporosis, ovarian and breast cancer in later life, as well as type II diabetes (Ip *et al.*, 2007). Ip *et al.* (2007) suggest that the protective factors of breastfeeding for mothers are also dose-related; that is, the longer a mother breastfeeds the better protection she receives, particularly for breast cancer. Ip *et al.* (2007) also suggest that early cessation of breastfeeding or not breastfeeding at all increases the risk of postnatal depression.

In addition, the WHO (2010a) suggest that breastfeeding helps mothers return to their pre-pregnancy weight more quickly by utilising the fat laid down in pregnancy for energy. Oxytocin, the hormone involved in the 'let-down' reflex, also causes contraction and involution of the uterus. Breastfeeding immediately following birth assists contraction of the uterus, encouraging placental separation and resulting in a possible reduction in postpartum blood loss (Leon-Cava *et al.*, 2002). A small study of 66 mothers in Sweden conducted by Jonas *et al.* (2008) concluded that breastfeeding also reduced both systolic and diastolic maternal blood pressure within two days of giving birth.

Many mothers are now aware that breastfeeding is associated with the above benefits. However, research continues to identify other diseases that breast-feeding may offer protection against. For example, in a large study of a million women, Liu *et al.* (2008) identified that the incidence of gall bladder disease increased by 8 per cent with each birth. However, the risk was reduced by 7 per cent for each year of breastfeeding. Pikwer *et al.* (2008) also suggested that women who breastfed for longer than 13 months were 50 per cent less likely to develop rheumatoid arthritis than those who had never breastfed and 25 per cent less likely if they breastfed for 1–12 months.

Other studies (Singhal, 2001; Armstrong and Reilly, 2002; Cregan *et al.*, 2002; Owen *et al.*, 2008; Khan *et al.*, 2009) have also demonstrated ongoing health benefits for those who were breastfed as infants, such as:

- reduced incidence of hypertension, cardiovascular disease, allergies and Crohn's disease;
- lower cholesterol;
- lower rates of obesity and type II diabetes;
- higher IQ.

Economic and environmental factors

As well as being safe and conferring health benefits, breastfeeding is also free and environmentally friendly. The Department of Health (DH, 2010c) estimates that it costs parents £45 per month to formula feed their infant. Leon-Cava *et al.* (2002) concluded, from their summary of the literature on the benefits of breastfeeding, that formula feeding could be financially 'prohibitive' or 'crippling' for some families, particularly if the infant becomes unwell and requires treatment, resulting in the mother being unable to go to work. It can also be said that the financial burden extends to society and the economy in general in terms of healthcare costs and absence from work.

In 2006, the NICE *Routine Postnatal Care of Women and Their Babies* costing report for promoting and increasing breastfeeding rates (NICE, 2006b, pp. 23–5), identified the following potential savings against the reduced incidence of otitis media, gastroenteritis and asthma. The estimates were based on a 10 per cent increase in breastfeeding rates based on an annual birth rate of 605,634:

- A 10 per cent increase in breastfeeding could lead to about 17,000 cases of otitis media being avoided at a saving of £509,000.
- A 10 per cent increase in breastfeeding could lead to almost 3,900 cases of gastroenteritis being avoided, at a saving of £2.6 million.
- A 10 per cent increase in breastfeeding could lead to over 1,500 cases of asthma being avoided, at a saving of £2.6 million.
- A 10 per cent increase in breastfeeding could lead to a reduction in the cost of teats and formula in hospitals of £102,000.
- NICE also acknowledged that savings could be made due to the health benefits of breastfeeding for mothers, but no estimation was provided.

Artificial feeding also has significant detrimental effects on the environment and contributes to global warming through cattle grazing and the consumption of fossil fuels in the production, distribution, disposal and waste of formula milk and packaging (WABA, 2005; Palmer, 2009), for example:

- Production of formula milk leads to deforestation of land required to graze cows, which also leads to increased sewage polluting rivers and ground water. Cow flatulence leads to approximately 20 per cent of global methane gas, which contributes to greenhouse gases and global warming.
- Production processes of plastic bottles and teats and other infant feeding equipment leads to increased carbon dioxide emissions and the plastics themselves contain toxins such as bisphenol-A (BPA). It is estimated that they can take up to 450 years to break down in landfill sites.
- Packaging of formula milk involves tins, paper and tetrapaks, most of which is not recycled.
- Transportation of formula milk and feeding equipment to distributors, and transportation of purchasers to buy the products uses valuable resources.

Because breastfeeding is available at source and on demand it uses none of the resources listed above and therefore does not create any pollution. Furthermore, lactational amenorrhoea in breastfeeding mothers helps reduce family sizes, which improves women's health, while reducing the production, distribution, disposal and waste of products associated with menstruation, such as sanitary towels and tampons.

Who breastfeeds?

Statistics provide healthcare professionals with important information about the characteristics of those who choose to breastfeed and for how long. This information enables the development of breastfeeding promotion programmes, policies and guidelines at national and local levels. On an individual level they also provide healthcare practitioners with an understanding of the reasons women make the choices they do. Dungy *et al.* (2008) suggest that knowledge and attitude can predict infant feeding intention and tools such as the Infant Feeding Attitude Scale (IFAS) could be used to develop and evaluate programmes aimed at promoting breastfeeding.

Despite the WHO (2002) recommendation for exclusive breastfeeding until the age of six months and to continue, alongside other foods, until the age of two years and beyond, breastfeeding rates in the UK continue to be among the lowest in Europe. The results of the *Infant Feeding Survey 2005* (Bolling *et al.*, 2007) demonstrated that the breastfeeding initiation rate for the UK was 78 per cent in England, 70 per cent in Scotland, 67 per cent in Wales and 63 per cent in Northern Ireland, followed by a rapid decline over the first few weeks. They found that 48 per cent of all mothers were breastfeeding at six weeks postpartum, and 25 per cent at six months. However, only 48 per cent of all mothers were exclusively breastfeeding at one week; only 25 per cent of these were still exclusively breastfeeding at six weeks and less than 1 per cent at six months.

The *Infant Feeding Survey 2005* (Bolling, *et al.*, 2007) is conducted every five years to provide estimates on incidence, prevalence and duration of breastfeeding. Between August and September 2005 a sample of 9,416 mothers from all birth registers in the UK were selected and returned completed questionnaires at three stages of the project. Stage one was conducted when the infant was four–ten weeks old, stage two at four–six months of age and stage three at eight–ten months of age.

The survey continually identified clear evidence of a relationship between breastfeeding and socio-demographic characteristics. Bolling *et al.* (2007) highlighted that increased rates of initiation of breastfeeding were associated with mothers who worked in managerial and professional occupations (*National Statistics Socio-economic Classification* system, 2005), who had the highest educational levels and were over the age of 30 years. In fact, mothers aged 35 years or over were found to be five times more likely to breastfeed than those under 20 years. These findings are supported by Bishop *et al.* (2008), who conducted a small questionnaire survey in a socio-economically deprived area in Northern Ireland. Using the Infant Feeding Assessment Tool they found similar results; older mothers who were in a relationship and had been breastfed themselves were more likely to breastfeed.

It is suggested that young mothers from socio-economically disadvantaged areas are less likely to breastfeed, due to embarrassment and misconceptions about breastfeeding, such as pain and lack of milk to satisfy the baby. Living in a bottle-feeding culture, they may not have witnessed breastfeeding first hand and may not have a role model (SACN, 2008b). They are also less likely to attend antenatal appointments and classes to receive education and information about breastfeeding than older mothers.

Mothers from all minority ethnic groups were also found to be more likely to breastfeed than white mothers. For example, between the years 2000 and 2005 there was an increase in initiating breastfeeding for white mothers from 68 per cent to 74 per cent, whereas the increase for Asian mothers was from 87 per cent to 94 per cent.

Returning to work was also highlighted as an influencing factor that reduced the duration of breastfeeding compared to those who did not.

It is of concern that the *Infant Feeding Survey 2005* (Bolling *et al.*, 2007) also demonstrated that not all mothers received appropriate support and advice from healthcare professionals, stating that only 79 per cent received information on the health benefits of breastfeeding; 68 per cent discussed feeding intention in the antenatal period (28 per cent at antenatal classes) and only seven out of ten mothers were shown how to put their infant to the breast in the first few days. This has major implications for healthcare professionals, and in particular midwives.

The common situations that lead to early weaning

Early introduction of solid food increases the risk of ill health for infants. Coinciding with changed advice from the WHO in 2002 and the DH (2003b, revised in 2008) regarding the timing of weaning from four to six months of age, the *Infant Feeding Survey 2005* (Bolling *et al.*, 2007) identified an improvement in the age when parents introduced solid foods into their infant's diet compared to 2000. In 2000, 85 per cent had introduced solid food before four months, whereas in 2005 this had decreased to 51 per cent. However, in 2005 only 2 per cent were following the recommendation to delay introducing solid food until six months of age. This trend was also reflected in a study conducted in Australia, by Retallack *et al.* (2008), who found that 40 per cent of infants under the age of four months had been introduced to solid foods, the majority of whom had been bottle-fed. Bolling *et al.* (2007) also identified that mothers in Scotland and Wales introduced solids earlier than those in England and Northern Ireland. Early weaning was also reported to be associated with lower social class groups and lower levels of education.

Bolling *et al.* (2007) identified that the decision of when to wean was influenced by the perception that the baby was not satisfied by milk alone (63 per cent), advice from family and friends (14 per cent) and previous experience (32 per cent). The DH (2010a, p. 21) also identified that some mothers decide to commence weaning for the following reasons:

- *Hunger*: Some parents often attribute night waking to hunger. However, this is most likely to be a growth spurt and increasing the number of breastfeeds for this period should be enough.
- *Energy needs*: Once the infant begins to move around, parents perceive that the energy requirements will not be met by milk alone.
- *Infant size and gender*: Boys are often perceived as requiring more food than girls, as are large infants. Some cultures perceive a big baby as a healthy baby.
- *Interest in food*: If the infant watches parents eat and mimics chewing, or dribbles, this can be perceived as readiness for solid food (see Chapter 9).
- *Previous experience*: If previous infants have been weaned early, it is likely to happen with subsequent children.

The DH (2010a) also suggests that mothers wean early because they do not understand the rationale for waiting for six months and they perceive the guideline as adaptable. They suggest that healthcare professionals have the same misconceptions and lack of understanding, viewing the recommendations as an 'ideal', and that some actively recommend introducing solids before six months. Also, infant food labels continue to recommend these products as suitable from the age of four months.

Another factor that was identified as a major influence in the timing of weaning was returning to work. Mothers who returned to work after six months, or not at all, introduced solids later than their counterparts who returned to work earlier. Other factors that were identified in the later introduction of solid foods were information provided by the health visitor (35 per cent), leaflets and other written material. However, these mothers tended to have higher levels of education.

As well as family and friends influencing decisions about weaning, culture also plays an important role. Some ethnic minority mothers introduce solids by two months of age for similar reasons as stated above, but with additional cultural issues. For example, some mothers thicken breast or formula milk with cornmeal, maize, cereal, rusks or semolina. There are also differences in the types of food introduced by different ethnic groups. Further details can be found in *Breastfeeding and Introducing Solid Foods: Consumer Insight Summary* (DH, 2010a).

The DH (2010a) also suggests that some mothers based their decision to wean their infants early on 'emotional' reasons, such as perceiving themselves to be a 'good mum' by preparing and providing food, excitement about reaching a new milestone in the infant's development, and being able to involve partners and relatives in infant feeding.

Introducing solid food will be discussed further in Chapter 9.

UNICEF UK Baby Friendly Initiative

In 1989 the WHO/UNICEF published the *Ten Steps to Successful Breastfeeding* in response to concerns about hospital practices; this was the forerunner to the WHO/UNICEF Baby Friendly Hospital Initiative, 1992. The aim of this initiative was to ensure that pregnant and breastfeeding women had access to high standards of care by supporting healthcare settings to implement best practice standards. In December 2010, changes to the UNICEF UK BFI's Hospital Initiative Programme were launched that reflected current knowledge to ensure it was fit for purpose (UNICEF, 2010e).

In 1998 the UNICEF UK BFI produced the *Seven Point Plan for the Protection, Promotion and Support of Breastfeeding in Community Healthcare Settings* which reflected the *Ten Steps*. This was updated in 2008 and renamed *The Seven Point Plan for Sustaining Breastfeeding in the Community* (www.babyfriendly.org.uk) – see Table 1.1 or Appendix 3 for further details. The BFI offers an assessment and accreditation process to acknowledge organisations that achieve these standards.

Implementation of the BFI best practice standards have been identified as a way to increase breastfeeding rates (Tappin *et al.*, 2001; Britten and Broadfoot, 2002; Broadfoot *et al.*, 2005a; Merten *et al.*, 2005). The *Ten Steps* and *Seven Point Plan* are seen as the hallmark of good practice and are recommended in the NICE guidelines, *Routine Postnatal Care of Women and their Babies* (2006a). Northern Ireland currently has 61.19 per cent of births in BFI-accredited hospitals, followed by Wales at 46.28 per cent, Scotland at 41.38 per cent and England at 10.12 per cent (UNICEF, 2010a).

Despite the success of these initiatives, concern has been expressed about the level of breastfeeding education for students in pre-registration programmes and why it is necessary for employers to provide additional education for registered midwives and health visitors within six months of employment to meet the BFI standards. This led, in 2002, to the development of the *Best Practice Standards for Higher Education Institutions* (UNICEF, 2008c).

The aim of education standards is to ensure that newly qualified midwives and health visitors are equipped with the basic knowledge and skills to support breastfeeding mothers effectively. Three standards and 18 outcomes were

TABLE 1.1 The *Ten Steps* and the *Seven Point Plan* (WHO/UNICEF)

Ten Steps		Seven Point Plan	
Step 1	Have a written breastfeeding policy that is routinely communicated to all healthcare staff	Point 1	Have a written breastfeeding policy that is routinely communicated to all healthcare staff
Step 2	Train all healthcare staff in skills necessary to implement the breastfeeding policy	Point 2	Train all healthcare staff in skills necessary to implement the policy
Step 3	Inform all pregnant women about the benefits and management of breastfeeding	Point 3	Inform all pregnant women about the benefits and management of breastfeeding
Step 4	Help mothers initiate breastfeeding soon after birth	Point 4	Support mothers to initiate and maintain breastfeeding
Step 5	Show mothers how to breastfeed and how to maintain lactation, even if they should be separated from their infants	Point 5	Encourage exclusive and continued breastfeeding, with appropriately timed introduction of complementary foods
Step 6	Give newborn infants no food or drink other than breastmilk, unless medically indicated	Point 6	Provide a welcoming atmosphere for breastfeeding families
Step 7	Practise rooming-in: allow mothers and infants to remain together 24 hours a day	Point 7	Promote co-operation between healthcare staff, breastfeeding support groups and the local community
Step 8	Encourage breastfeeding on demand		
Step 9	Give no artificial teats or dummies to breastfeeding infants		
Step 10	Identify sources of national and local support for breastfeeding and refer mothers to these prior to discharge from hospital		

Source: www.babyfriendly.org.uk (updated 2010).

developed, based on the *Ten Steps to Successful Breastfeeding* and *Seven Point Plan* (UNICEF, 1998), to be introduced into the curriculum and successfully achieved at the point of registration as a midwife or health visitor. The intention was to 'equip students to enable and support parents to make informed choices about infant feeding and to deliver effective care for breastfeeding mothers and babies' (UNICEF, 2002, p. 2).

The education standards and outcomes involve fundamental and basic knowledge about the normal anatomy of the breasts, the physiology of lactation and the practical skills of breastfeeding, incorporating research-based evidence and consideration of the psycho-social factors that influence successful breastfeeding (UNICEF, 2002) (see Appendix 1 for further details).

In a single-site case study in one of the first BFI-accredited pre-registration midwifery programmes in the UK, Pollard (2010) stated that student midwives reported feeling theoretically prepared for practice-based placements for their level of education and graduates of the programme also reported feeling confident at the point of registration to support and advise breastfeeding mothers. She also found that the accreditation process promoted a consistent approach to teaching and learning strategies, as well as content, within the curriculum. Furthermore, students believed it enhanced their employability prospects.

More recently, the UNICEF UK BFI developed standards for neonatal units (see Appendix 5 for further details) to provide guidance on best practice for breastfeeding infants who are preterm or ill, and are separated from their mothers. These standards are in addition to best practice standards for maternity units. The BFI does not have an accreditation process specifically for neonatal units; however, it is expected that all neonatal staff will be trained to support breastfeeding mothers. These standards will be discussed further in Chapter 7.

Global and national strategies

The WHO Code

The WHO (1981) developed the *International Code of Marketing of Breast-milk Substitutes*, known as the 'Code', to protect and promote breastfeeding and ensure the proper use of breastmilk substitutes. It is a World Health Assembly (WHA) resolution aimed at tackling a global health problem (Palmer, 2009). Some of the requirements are:

- all formula milk labels should state the benefits of breastfeeding and the risks of formula feeding;
- there should be no promotion of breastmilk substitutes (this includes follow-on formulas, and any solid foods or drinks sold for infants under the age of six months);
- no free samples of breastmilk substitutes are to be given to pregnant women;
- no free samples or subsidised substitutes are to be given to health workers or healthcare facilities;
- there should be no gifts for healthcare workers;

Box 1.1 UNICEF UK BFI *Best Practice Standards for Higher Education Institutions*

1   Understand the importance of breastfeeding and the consequences of not breastfeeding in terms of health outcomes.
2   Have developed an in-depth knowledge of the physiology of lactation and be able to apply this in practical situations.
3   Be able to recognise effective positioning, attachment and suckling and to empower mothers to develop the skills necessary for them to achieve these for themselves.
4   Be able to demonstrate knowledge of the principles of hand expression and have the ability to teach these to mothers.
5   Understand the potential impact of delivery room practices on the well-being of mother and baby and on the establishment of breastfeeding in particular.
6   Understand why it is important for mothers to keep their babies near them.
7   Understand the principle of demand feeding and be able to explain its importance in relation to the establishment and maintenance of lactation.
8   Be equipped to provide parents with accurate, evidence-based information about activities which may have an impact on breastfeeding.
9   Understand the importance of exclusive breastfeeding for the first six months of life and possess the knowledge and skills to enable mothers to achieve this.
10 Understand the importance of timely introduction of complementary foods and of continuing breastfeeding during the weaning period, into the second year of life and beyond.
11 Understand the importance of community support for breastfeeding and demonstrate an awareness of the role of community-based support networks, both in supporting women to breastfeed and as a resource for health professionals.
12 Be able to support mothers who are separated from their babies (e.g. on admission to SCBU, when returning to work) to initiate and/or maintain their lactation and to feed their babies optimally.
13 Be able to demonstrate a knowledge of alternative methods of infant feeding and care which may be used where breastfeeding is not possible and which will enhance the likelihood of a later transition to breastfeeding.
14 Identify babies who require a managed approach to feeding and describe appropriate care.
15 Know about the common complications of breastfeeding, how these arise and how women may be helped to overcome them.

16 Understand the limited number of situations in which exclusive breastfeeding is not possible and be able to support mothers in partial breastfeeding or artificial feeding in these circumstances.

17 Appreciate the main differences between the WHO *International Code of Marketing of Breast-milk Substitutes* and the relevant current UK legislation and understand the relevance of the Code to their own work situation.

18 Be thoroughly conversant with the BFI best practice standards, understand the rationale behind them and what the BFI seeks to achieve through them and be equipped to implement them in their own workplace, with appropriate support from colleagues.

Box 1.2 UNICEF UK BFI *Best Practice Standards for Establishing and Maintaining Lactation and Breastfeeding in Neonatal Units*

1 Have a written (neonatal unit) breastfeeding policy which is routinely communicated to all staff.

2 Educate all healthcare staff in the skills necessary to implement the policy.

3 Inform all parents of the benefits of breastmilk and breastfeeding babies in the neonatal unit.

4 Facilitate skin-to-skin (kangaroo care) between mother and baby.

5 Support mothers to initiate and maintain lactation through expression of breastmilk.

6 Support mothers to establish and maintain breastfeeding.

7 Encourage exclusive breastmilk feeding.

8 Avoid the use of teats or dummies for breastfed babies unless clinically indicated.

9 Promote breastfeeding support through local and national networks.

Source: www.babyfriendly.org.uk/pdfs/neonatal_standards.pdf (see Appendix 5 for further details).

- labels on products should not idealise formula feeding and should be written in an appropriate language;
- all information for healthcare workers should be factual and scientific.

It has been suggested that the Code removes choice from mothers, but instead the Code aims to improve choice by ensuring that advertising provides factual information for mothers on which to base their choices, rather than biased information to sell the product. Although formula milk companies state that breast is best on their products, they do not provide information on the dangers of not breastfeeding. They also use persuasive language to suggest that formula milk is as 'good' as breastmilk when this is not possible.

The aim of adhering to the Code is to provide mothers with evidence-based information so that they can make an informed choice about infant feeding and to protect against misleading marketing. UNICEF UK BFI (2008a) identified marketing activities of artificial milk companies and hospital practices as major reasons for the decline in breastfeeding in the twentieth century. It is important that healthcare professionals do not accept gifts or samples from formula milk companies (which often include pens, diary covers, calendars and obstetric calculators), as these products are part of the marketing strategy and accepting them suggests that healthcare professionals are endorsing the product.

However, if a mother chooses to formula feed her infant, all healthcare professionals should be equipped with up-to-date, factual and scientific information about the artificial milks available. Material available in healthcare journals is often intended for marketing purposes and therefore does not give all the facts. To combat this, many healthcare providers now invite formula milk company representatives to present new, factual information to designated members of staff so that it can be disseminated in an appropriate and unbiased way. Healthcare workers must be objective when supporting mothers with formula feeding and should not be promoting one brand over another (NMC, 2008).

The Code was not fully adopted by UK in law; instead, the government passed the *1995 Infant Formula and Follow-on Formula Regulations* (DH, 2010b). However, many healthcare settings that work to promote and protect breastfeeding and reduce inappropriate breastmilk substitute marketing have adopted the Code as part of their professional standards. Other professional and lay organisations have done the same, for example:

- UNICEF UK Baby Friendly Initiative;
- Baby Milk Action (BMA);
- International Baby Food Action Network (IBFAN);
- *Breastfeeding Manifesto* (BFM);
- Baby Feeding Law Group (BFLG).

TABLE 1.2 Differences between the WHO Code and UK law

WHO Code	UK law
No advertising or promotion anywhere	Advertising allowed in healthcare system
No free samples or gifts to mothers/ the public	Gifts to the public allowed, if not designed to promote sales
No free or subsidised supplies to hospitals unless for research	Less clear specification
No free gifts to healthcare workers; information must be scientific and factual	Gifts to healthcare workers allowed; information not strictly controlled
No contact between mothers and company representatives	Contact between mothers and company representatives allowed if instigated by the mother – carelines etc.

Source: UNICEF (2008a, p. 71).

In 2007, the UK Minister for Public Health established a review of the *Infant Formula and Follow-on Formula Regulations* to reduce the confusion for parents between infant formula for exclusive feeding of infants during the first months of life and follow-on formula for infants aged six months and over (DH, 2010b). They made the following recommendations:

- that manufacturers should make changes to advertising to make it clear that follow-on formula is intended for infants over six months by clearly representing the age of the infants in the adverts;
- that any problems encountered with the enforcement of the regulations should be addressed accordingly.

The full report can be found on the Department of Health website (www.dh.gov.uk).

Innocenti Declaration

The *Innocenti Declaration on the Protection, Promotion and Support of Breast-feeding* (WHO, 1990) was developed by WHO and UNICEF policy makers in 1990 and adopted in the UK and many other countries. It acknowledged the importance of exclusive breastfeeding for the first six months of life and its continuance thereafter alongside the introduction of solid foods. At the time it was apparent that there needed to be a change in some countries away from a bottle-feeding culture to a breastfeeding culture, which could only be achieved by removing obstacles to breastfeeding within healthcare systems, the work-place and society in general and, in doing so, increasing women's confidence in their ability to breastfeed. The declaration made the following recommendations:

- Women should be adequately nourished.
- Women should have access to family planning services to increase birth intervals and improve their health.
- All governments should develop a national breastfeeding policy and set appropriate targets that can be monitored.
- Breastfeeding policies should be integrated into other health and development policies.
- All governments should train healthcare staff to be able to implement the policies.
- National breastfeeding advisers should be appointed.
- Healthcare facilities should adhere to the WHO/UNICEF *Ten Steps to Successful Breastfeeding*.
- All governments should take cognisance of the *International Code of Marketing of Breast-milk Substitutes* and the WHA resolutions.
- All governments should enact legislation to protect breastfeeding mothers.

Activity

It is interesting to see how far the UK has come since the *Innocenti Declaration* in 1990. Identify some of the more recent and relevant policy documents that have recognised the need to promote breastfeeding to reduce health inequalities in your country of practice.

National strategies

In recent years in the UK, there have been numerous developments in national policy that address most of the recommendations from the *Innocenti Declaration*; however, to date the UK has not fully implemented the *International Code of Marketing of Breast-milk Substitutes*. Below are several examples of policy to promote, support and protect breastfeeding but this list is by no means exhaustive.

In 2001 in the UK, the Scientific Advisory Committee on Nutrition (SACN) concluded that there was enough evidence to support the WHO (2002) guidance to promote exclusive breastfeeding for the first six months of life. In 2003 the Department of Health revised its guidelines to recommend:

- breastmilk as the best form of nutrition for infants;
- exclusive breastfeeding for the first six months of an infant's life;
- six months as the recommended age for the introduction of solid foods;
- breastfeeding (and/or infant formula) should be continued beyond the first six months, alongside appropriate solid foods.

In 2006, 'Healthy Start' replaced the Welfare Food Scheme. It was aimed at disadvantaged and low-income households in England, Scotland, Wales and Northern Ireland, providing vouchers for free milk, fruit and vegetables and vitamins for pregnant women and parents of young children. Those on jobseeker's allowance, income support or child tax credit, or under the age of 18 years, are eligible for Healthy Start benefits. Further details can be found at www.healthystart.nhs.uk. The aim of this initiative was to encourage contact with healthcare professionals who could provide advice on pregnancy, breastfeeding, weaning and healthy eating in general.

Also in 2006, the National Institute for Health and Clinical Excellence (NICE) produced guidance on *Routine Postnatal Care of Women and their Babies*. While suggesting that further research is required into the cost-effectiveness of the BFI, the postnatal care guideline recommended that 'All healthcare providers (hospitals and community) should implement an externally evaluated structured programme that encourages breastfeeding, using the Baby Friendly Initiative as a minimum standard' (2006a, p. 38).

The Department of Health went on to request that NICE produce further public health guidance to assist health professionals to improve the nutrition of pregnant and breastfeeding mothers and children in low-income house-holds and other disadvantaged groups. In March 2008, NICE published *Public Health Guidance 11* (www.nice.org.uk/PH011), which made 22 recommendations to support improvement in the nutrition of pregnant and breastfeeding mothers from low-income households. It was aimed at health professionals working with women and young children; child health com-missioners, managers of maternity and child health services, community health partnership directors and public, community, voluntary and private sector organisations.

In addition, each country in the UK has developed its own infant feeding strategy and specific guidance in relation to breastfeeding. The following are some examples of these initiatives:

- In England, the *NHS Priorities and Planning Framework 2003–6* explored local plans to improve breastfeeding rates, with a particular focus on disadvantaged groups. A target of an increase in breastfeeding of 2 per cent per year was set. Three times a year Primary Care Trusts are required to submit data on initiation rates of breastfeeding and prevalence of breastfeeding at six to eight weeks (further information can be found at www.dh.gov.uk). Also, in 2008 the government pledged £2 million to help hospitals improve breastfeeding rates and achieve BFI accreditation.

- In Wales, *Investing in a Better Start: Promoting breastfeeding in Wales* (2001) was developed to support the increase in initiation and duration of breastfeeding, and in 2003 a *National Breastfeeding Strategy Implementation Group* was established.

- In Scotland, *The Scottish Breastfeeding Group*, now called the *Scottish Infant Feeding Advisory Network* was established to disseminate good practice and a national breastfeeding adviser was appointed. The HEAT (Health improvement, Efficiency, Access, Treatment) targets were agreed between the Scottish Executive Health Department and each NHS Health Board to reflect the government's key priorities. One of these HEAT targets was to increase the proportion of newborn children exclusively breastfed at six to eight weeks from 26.6 per cent in 2006/07 to 33.3 per cent in 2010/11.

- In 2002, a regional breastfeeding coordinator was appointed to promote and advise on the *Breastfeeding Strategy for Northern Ireland*. The Health Promotion Agency has also developed a variety of resources for parents and professionals.

Activity

Locate your local breastfeeding strategy and critically evaluate it to see if it reflects the national breastfeeding strategy.

- Have local breastfeeding targets been set?
- How are breastfeeding rates monitored?

Breastfeeding in public

Women have consistently reported negative attitudes and sometimes abuse directed at them when breastfeeding in public; and on occasion they have been removed from public areas or transport. In 2005, The Breastfeeding (Scotland) Act was passed, which made it an offence to prevent a person feeding milk by bottle or breast to an infant in a public place where the infant is legally entitled to be. Milk referred to breast, formula or cow's milk. Anyone who deliberately prevents a child being breast- or bottle-fed is guilty of an offence that could result in a fine. It was also intended that the Act would encourage, support and promote breastfeeding in Scotland by addressing negative attitudes.

Following this, in April 2009, the UK government presented an Equality Bill proposing that it was unlawful to prevent a woman from breastfeeding her baby in public. It was referred to as 'maternity' discrimination, which caused some confusion initially as this may only relate to six months before or after the birth and would therefore possibly not legally protect mothers breastfeeding for six months and beyond. It was amended to clarify that it meant mothers breastfeeding at any time.

The *Infant Feeding Survey 2005* (Bolling *et al.*, 2007) stated that half of mothers who breastfeed had done so in public, this number rising to all mothers if they fed until six months. Only 3 per cent of mothers had been stopped or asked not to breastfeed in public, but 13 per cent had been made to feel uncomfortable. Interestingly, the survey identified mothers in Scotland as having more positive breastfeeding experiences in public.

Concluding comments

It is clear from the evidence that breastfeeding is essential in reducing health inequalities in mothers and infants in the UK. Despite this, mothers continue to face barriers that either discourage them from commencing breastfeeding or lead to early cessation of breastfeeding. Healthcare professionals need to be aware of the challenges mothers face in society and be equipped with the knowledge and skills to support them to overcome these barriers and confidently to provide consistent information to manage these challenges as they arise. There is a wealth of information available to both mothers and healthcare professionals today, particularly online, and access is now available to most people. Developing knowledge and skills to support breastfeeding mothers will be discussed further in Chapter 11.

Practice questions

1   In your area of practice, how and when do you inform mothers about the benefits of breastfeeding and the dangers of not breastfeeding?
2   Are there services targeted at the socio-economic characteristics of mothers in your area of practice? How do women find out about available services?
3   Go back and read the *Ten Steps* and *Seven Point Plan* in Table 1.1. Are these standards implemented in your area of practice? If not, why not?
4   In relation to marketing of formula milk, does your area of practice comply with the WHO Code? How do you find out about new information on formula milk?
5   Has your university integrated the BFI educational outcomes into the pre-registration programmes?
6   If yes, what difference do you think this has made to your practice?
7   If no, what advantages do you think accreditation would bring to the programmes and to practice?

Resources

*   Baby Feeding Law Group (BFLG)
        www.babyfeedinglawgroup.org.uk
*   Baby Milk Action (BMA)
        www.babymilkaction.org
*   *Best Beginnings: From Bump to Breastfeeding* DVD
        www.bestbeginnings.org.uk
*   *Breastfeeding Manifesto* (BFM)
        www.breastfeedingmanifesto.org.uk
*   Healthy Start
        www.healthystart.nhs.uk
*   International Baby Food Action Network (IBFAN)
        www.ibfan.org
*   Scientific Advisory Committee on Nutrition (SACN)
        www.sacn.gov.uk
*   UNICEF UK Baby Friendly Initiative
        www.babyfriendly.org.uk

Chapter 2 **Anatomy and physiology of lactation**

- Learning outcomes
- Relevant anatomy and physiology
- The physiology of lactation
- Constituents of breastmilk
- Neonatal adaptation to life
- Concluding comments
- True or false quiz
- Further reading

It is essential for healthcare professionals to have a sound knowledge of the external and internal anatomy of the breast, as well as the physiology of lactation, to support mothers effectively to feel confident about positioning and attachment, hand expression and the management of common problems. This chapter begins with an introduction to breast development in puberty, pregnancy and lactation and goes on to discuss the anatomy of the breast and the physiology of lactation. The previous chapter discussed the benefits of breastmilk in promoting good health and reducing health inequalities; this chapter will move on to discuss the properties of breastmilk that make it the ideal form of nutrition for human infants. Finally, production of breastmilk will not be continued without effective removal of breastmilk from the breast and therefore it is crucial that healthcare professionals have a clear understanding of the mechanism of suckling and adaptation to life to teach mothers to recognise appropriate feeding behaviour.

Learning outcomes

By the end of this chapter you will be able to:

- understand breast development in pregnancy and lactation;
- describe the anatomy of the breast;
- understand the physiology of lactation;
- describe the constituents and value of colostrums and breastmilk;
- demonstrate an understanding of the mechanism of infant suckling.

Mapping the UNICEF UK BFI educational outcomes

1   Understand the importance of breastfeeding and the consequences of not breastfeeding in terms of health outcomes.
2   Have developed an in-depth knowledge of the physiology of lactation and be able to apply this in practical situations.
3   Be able to recognise effective positioning, attachment and suckling and to empower mothers to develop the skills necessary for them to achieve these for themselves.

Relevant anatomy and physiology

Mammogenesis

Mammogenesis is the term used for the development of the mammary glands or breasts, which occurs in five stages:

- embryogenesis;
- puberty;
- pregnancy;
- lactation;
- involution.

Embryogenesis

Breast development begins at about the fourth week of gestation in both male and female fetuses. By 12 to 16 weeks the development of the nipple and areola is evident. The lactiferous ducts open into the mammary pit, which elevates to become the nipple and areola (Walker, 2002). After birth some neonates born at term secrete a fluid referred to as *'witch's milk'* (not known in premature infants), due to the influence of the maternal hormones associated with milk production (Lawrence and Lawrence, 2005).

Interesting fact

Witch's milk is present in both sexes and can continue up to two months of age. The name 'witch's milk' is derived from folklore, where it was thought to be a source of nourishment for witches' familiars and was taken from sleeping babies.

Puberty

There is no further breast development until puberty, when increasing levels of oestrogen and progesterone lead to growth of lactiferous ducts, alveoli, the nipple and areola (Stables and Rankin, 2010). The increase in breast size is due to the deposition of adipose tissue (Geddes, 2007b).

Pregnancy and lactogenesis

For many women breast changes can be one of the first signs of pregnancy. At about the sixth week of pregnancy, oestrogen promotes the growth of the lactiferous ducts, while progesterone, prolactin and human placental lactogen (HPL) leads to proliferation and enlargement of the alveoli; women describe a 'tingling' sensation, sensitivity and heaviness of their breasts (Stables and Rankin, 2010). With the increasing blood supply, veins become visible on the surface of the breasts. At 12 weeks there is greater pigmentation to the areola and nipples due to increased melanocytes, and they become red/brown in colour. The *Montgomery's tubercles* also become more prominent and begin to excrete a serous lubricant to protect the nipple and areola. At approximately 16 weeks, colostrum is produced (lactogenesis I) under the influence of prolactin and HPL, but complete milk production is suppressed by the increased levels of oestrogen and progesterone (Lawrence and Lawrence, 2005). However, some women may find they secrete a clear fluid prior to this. At approximately 24 weeks, the secondary areola is formed around the areola (Stables and Rankin, 2010). Lactation is considered to be the point where breasts have achieved their full development (Walker, 2002).

Involution

Involution occurs when weaning takes place and milk is no longer removed from the breast. Prolactin production is no longer stimulated and there is milk stasis and subsequent build-up of feedback inhibitor of lactation (FIL), which inhibits further milk synthesis. The secretory epithelial cells die (apoptosis), are reabsorbed and the breasts return to the pre-pregnant size by approximately 15 months (Kent, 2007).

As the infant is introduced to solid food, the composition and volume of breastmilk changes from an average of 759ml per day to 95–315ml per day at 15 months of age. There is also a decrease in glucose and minerals and an increase in fat, lactose, protein and sodium (Kent, 2007), giving the milk a more salty taste.

External structure of the breast

The breasts, or mammary glands, are hemispherical in shape with an axillary tail and are situated on each side of the anterior chest wall (see Figure 2.1). They extend from the second to the sixth rib, from the sternum to the axilla (the *Tail of Spence*), over the pectoralis muscles. They are supported by fibrous connective tissue called Cooper's ligaments. Every mother's breasts vary in size; this is determined by the amount of fatty tissue, not glandular tissue. Size is not an indicator of milk storage capacity. Each mother's storage capacity is also variable but, despite this, over a 24-hour period, all lactating mothers produce a similar amount of breastmilk (average 798g/24 hours) (Kent *et al.*, 2006). The main difference will be noted in feeding patterns and those mothers with lower storage capacity will breastfeed more frequently than those with higher storage capacity, thus supporting the argument for baby-led feeding.

At the midpoint on the exterior surface lies the *areola*, a pigmented area. On average the areola measures 15mm in diameter; however, every woman's areola differs in size and colour. The Montgomery's tubercles open into the areola and secrete a protective oily secretion to lubricate the nipple during breastfeeding. The dark area of the areola is thought to assist the baby to find the nipple at birth and the scent is also thought to help attract the infant to suckle at the breast (Schaal *et al.*, 2005; Geddes, 2007b). The *nipple* is a sensitive erectile structure that contains smooth muscle, collagen and elastic connective tissue found in both circular and radial formations. Erection of the nipple is stimulated by tactile and autonomic sympathetic responses. It lies at the centre of the areola, from where breastmilk is ejected on demand. Stimulation of the nipple causes milk ejection via the hypothalamus, which stimulates oxytocin release from the posterior pituitary gland (Walker, 2002).

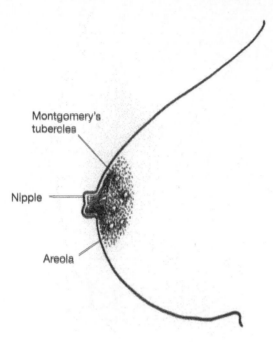

Montgomery's tubercles

Nipple

Areola

FIGURE 2.1 The external structure of the breast

Internal structure of the lactating breast

Until recently, the internal anatomy of the breast was based on wax casts from dissections of cadavers by Sir Astley Cooper in 1840. In 2005, Ramsay *et al.* conducted research using ultrasound imaging and described a number of differences in the structure of the breast.

The *lactiferous ducts* were previously thought to lead to the lactiferous sinus; however, Ramsay *et al.* (2005) found that the ducts branched off within the *areola* approximately 5–8mm from the nipple, closer to the nipple than previously thought, and did not demonstrate evidence of sinuses. The *lactiferous ducts* are small (mean diameter 2mm), superficial and easy to compress (see Figure 2.2). The authors of this study suggest that the ducts are responsible for transportation of the milk rather than storage. They also found that the network of milk ducts is not homogeneous as previously suggested (Figure 2.3 identifies the changes). Ramsay *et al.* (2005) found that there were 4–18 (av. 9) main milk ducts.

The breast is shaped by the fat and glandular tissue, which is inseparable except subcutaneously where there is only fat (Nickell and Skelton, 2005). The ratio of glandular to fat tissue increases to a ratio of 2:1 in the lactating breast, compared to 1:1 in non-lactating women, and 65 per cent of the glandular tissue is located within 30mm from the base of the nipple (Hilton, 2008).

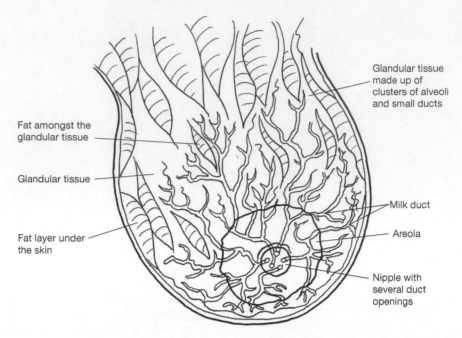

Glandular tissue made up of clusters of alveoli and small ducts

Fat amongst the glandular tissue

Glandular tissue

Fat layer under the skin

Milk duct

Areola

Nipple with several duct openings

FIGURE 2.2 The internal anatomy of the lactating breast

Source: adapted from © UNICEF UK BFI.

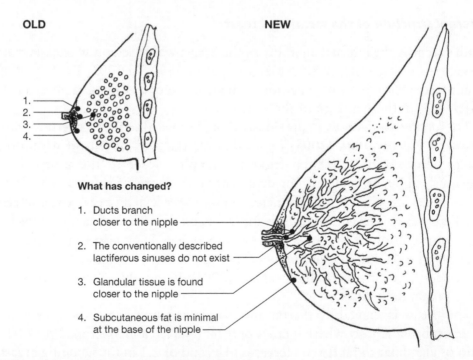

OLD

NEW

1.
2.
3.
4.

What has changed?

1. Ducts branch closer to the nipple

2. The conventionally described lactiferous sinuses do not exist

3. Glandular tissue is found closer to the nipple

4. Subcutaneous fat is minimal at the base of the nipple

FIGURE 2.3 The changed anatomy of the breast

Source: adapted from © Medela, AG, Switzerland.

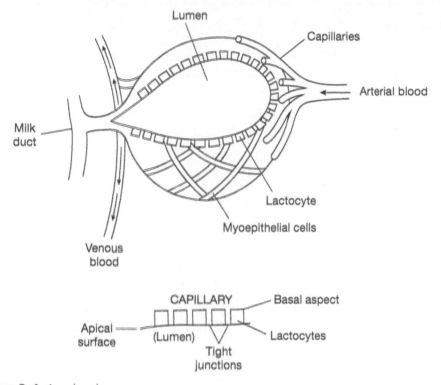

FIGURE 2.4 An alveolus

Source: adapted from Berry *et al.* (2007).

Numerous *alveoli* (10–100) (see Figure 2.4) cluster to form lobules, which are grouped into lobes. They are often described as being like a bunch of grapes. The alveoli consist of a single layer of the milk-producing *lactocytes* (*secretory epithelium*), which are surrounded by a network of capillaries. Lactocytes line the lumen of the alveoli and are cuboidal in shape if full, and columnar if empty. They are connected to each other and regulate the composition of breastmilk for collection in the lumen of the alveoli. It is this shape or fullness of the lactocyte that controls synthesis of breastmilk. If the lactocyte becomes too full and the shape distorts, the prolactin receptor sites do not function, leading to decreased milk synthesis (vanVeldhuizen-Staas, 2007). Once emptied, the lactocytes resume the normal columnar shape and milk synthesis can recommence. Tight junctions connect these cells and are closed in the first few days of lactation, preventing the passage of molecules through the space. The portion of the lactocytes facing the lumen is called the *apical surface*; the outer aspect is *basal*. Milk secretion occurs at the apical surface, whereas the basal aspect of the cell is responsible for the selection and synthesis of substrates from the blood (Geddes, 2007b).

> ### Key fact
>
> Breasts should be effectively emptied on a regular basis, either by suckling or expression, otherwise the shape of the lactocytes distorts and milk production ceases.

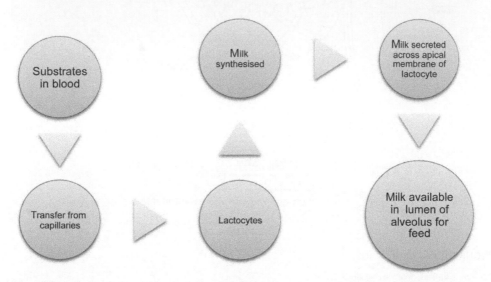

FIGURE 2.5 Pathway for the synthesis of breastmilk

The alveoli are surrounded by *myoepithelial cells*, which, under the influence of oxytocin, contract to expel the breastmilk from the lumen of the *alveolus* along the lactiferous ducts to the awaiting infant (see Figure 2.5). Multiple milk ejections occur during a breastfeed or expression of milk, with a range of 0–9 (Geddes, 2007b).

Blood, nerves and lymphatic system

The breasts are highly vascular; 60 per cent of the blood supply is via the internal mammary artery and 30 per cent via the lateral thoracic artery. Venous drainage is via the mammary and axillary veins. The lymphatic system drains excess fluid from the tissue spaces into the axillary nodes and mammary nodes (Geddes, 2007b).

The skin is supplied by branches of the thoracic nerves; the nipple and areola by the autonomic nervous system. The nerve supply is mainly from branches of the fourth, fifth and sixth intercostal nerves. The fourth intercostal nerve becomes superficial at the areola where it divides into five branches. Trauma, such as breast surgery, to this nerve may lead to loss of sensation (Walker, 2002; Geddes, 2007a).

The physiology of lactation

Lactogenesis is the initiation of milk production. There are three phases of lactogenesis. The first two phases are hormonally driven or *neuroendocrine* responses (interaction between the nervous system and the endocrine system) and occur whether the mother intends to breastfeed or not; the third is *autocrine* (a cell secretes a hormone chemical that acts on itself) or by local control.

Neuroendocrine control

Lactogenesis I is thought to occur at around 16 weeks' gestation when colostrum is produced by lactocytes under neuroendocrine control. Prolactin, although present during pregnancy, is inhibited by the increased levels of progesterone and oestrogen as well as HPL and prolactin-inhibiting factor (PIF) and therefore milk production is suppressed (Walker, 2010). However, some mothers may leak colostrum or choose to express colostrum from 36 weeks (see Chapter 6, 'Diabetes', page 112).

Lactogenesis II is the onset of milk production. It occurs following expulsion of the placenta and membranes, which results in a sudden drop in progesterone, oestrogen, HPL and PIF (neuroendocrine control). Prolactin levels increase and bind with prolactin receptors in the walls of the lactocytes, which are no longer deactivated by HPL and PIF, and begin milk synthesis (Lawrence and Lawrence, 2005). Skin-to-skin contact at birth with the baby stimulates the production of prolactin and oxytocin. Early and regular breastfeeding inhibits the production of PIF and stimulates production of prolactin. Mothers should

---

Key fact

Lactogenesis II may be delayed in mothers with type 1 diabetes, possibly due to the initial imbalance in insulin levels required for lactation, and those with retained placental products due to prolonged production of progesterone. Therefore, prolonged skin-to-skin contact from birth should be encouraged for uninterrupted access to the breast. If the infant does not suckle, regular hand expression will be required to stimulate milk production.

---

be encouraged to commence breastfeeding as soon as possible following birth to stimulate milk production and to provide infants with colostrum (see 'Colostrum' on page 34) (Czank *et al.*, 2007; Walker, 2010).

Lactogenesis II commences 30–40 hours after birth, but mothers do not feel the milk 'coming in' until about 2–3 days after birth. The increase in milk production is associated with the closure of the tight junctions between the lactocytes (Czank *et al.*, 2007).

Prolactin

Prolactin is the hormone essential in the establishment and maintenance of breastmilk production and is highest following the delivery of the placenta and membranes (200µg l) but gradually reduces by six months postpartum (80µg l) (Cox *et al.*, 1996). It is released into the blood from the anterior pituitary gland, in responses to suckling or nipple stimulation, and primes and stimulates the prolactin receptor sites on the walls of the lactocytes to synthesise milk (Czank *et al.*, 2007). The prolactin receptor sites regulate the secretion of breastmilk. When the alveoli are full of milk, the walls expand and change shape, affecting the prolactin receptor sites; ultimately, prolactin is unable to enter the cells and the milk production rate decreases. As the milk is emptied from the alveolus, its normal shape is returned and prolactin will bind to the receptor site, increasing milk production (vanVeldhuizen-Staas, 2007). Prolactin is also secreted during breastfeeding and is at its highest rate 45 minutes after a feed. Prolactin levels peak at night (circadian rhythm) and therefore night feeds must be encouraged to promote milk production (Walker, 2010).

> **Key fact**
>
> The prolactin receptor theory suggests that frequent milk removal in the early days increases the number of prolactin receptor sites 'switched on', thus improving milk production.

Oxytocin

Oxytocin is released from the posterior pituitary gland and stimulates contraction of the *myoepithelial cells* surrounding the alveoli to eject milk through the lactiferous ducts. This is commonly referred to as the let-down, oxytocin or ejection reflex. It causes shortening of the lactiferous ducts, to increase the intraductal mammary pressure and thus to facilitate milk ejection.

TABLE 2.1 The influence of other hormones on lactation

Hormones	Function
Glucocorticoids	Essential for mammary development in pregnancy, onset of lactogenesis II and maintenance of lactogenesis (galactopoesis).
Growth hormone	Essential for the maintenance of lactation by regulating metabolism.
Insulin	Ensures nutrients are readily available for milk synthesis.
Placental lactogen	Produced by the placenta and stimulates mammary development and growth, but is not involved in lactogenesis I or II.
Progesterone	Inhibits lactogenesis II during pregnancy by suppressing the prolactin receptor sites in the lactocytes. Once lactation is established, progesterone has little effect on breastmilk supply and therefore the progesterone-only contraceptive pill may be used by breastfeeding mothers (Czank *et al.*, 2007).
Thyroxin	Assists the breasts to be responsive to growth hormone and prolactin.

Some women feel a 'tingling' sensation in the breast and uterine contractions with increased bleeding per vagina within the first few days after birth. Some also describe feeling thirsty, flushing and becoming sleepy. Oxytocin, often called the 'love hormone', reduces cortisol levels, resulting in a relaxing effect, reducing anxiety and blood pressure, and promoting maternal behaviour (Moberg, 2003). The let-down reflex is controlled in the first few days following birth by the neonate suckling at the breast and also by the mother seeing, touching, hearing and smelling her baby (Prime *et al.*, 2007). As the infant becomes older the let-down reflex may be triggered by thinking about feeding the baby or hearing another baby cry. Ramsay *et al.* (2005) found that 75 per cent of breastfeeding mothers experience more than one let-down reflex per feed (av. 2.5) and that 33 per cent of infants end the feed after the first let-down reflex. The let-down reflex can, however, be inhibited by stress and anxiety (Prime *et al.*, 2007).

It is thought that suckling in the neonate is optimal at 45 minutes following birth and declines within two to three hours in line with the physiological reduction in neonatal adrenaline levels at birth (Stables and Rankin, 2010). It is therefore important that mothers and infants are able to have skin-to-skin contact for a minimum of one hour following birth to encourage early feeding, which ensures that prolactin is released, leading to the commencement of lactogenesis II (UNICEF, 2010e). Other factors thought to interfere with lactogenesis are retained placenta, Sheehan's syndrome or pituitary shock, breast surgery, type I diabetes, preterm delivery, obesity and stress. These issues will be addressed in Chapters 6 and 7.

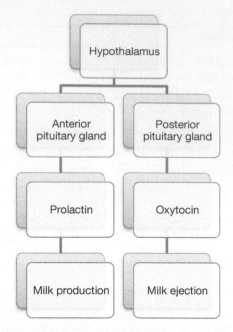

FIGURE 2.6 The neuroendocrine response

Practice recommendations

- Encourage skin-to-skin contact for a minimum of one hour following birth.
- Encourage suckling at the breast as soon after birth as possible to stimulate production of prolactin.
- Encourage regular breastfeeding and promote night feeds when levels of prolactin are highest. If this is not possible, regular expression of breastmilk is required.
- Avoid separation of the mother and infant and promote 'rooming-in'.
- Create a relaxed environment for feeding or expressing because stress inhibits the release of oxytocin.

Autocrine control

Lactogenesis III indicates the autocrine regulation where supply and demand regulate milk production. As well as the neuroendocrine response described earlier, milk supply is also controlled at the breast by milk removal through autocrine or local control. By studying milk production in goats, the Hannah Institute, Ayr, identified a whey protein called the feedback inhibitor of lactation (FIL), secreted by the lactocytes, which regulated milk production at a local level (Wilde *et al.*, 1995; Knight *et al.*, 1998). As the alveoli distend, there is a build-up of FIL and milk synthesis is inhibited. When the breastmilk is effectively removed and the concentrations of FIL reduce, milk synthesis resumes. This is a local mechanism and can occur in one or both breasts. It exerts a negative feedback response to inhibit milk production when there is ineffective removal of the breastmilk from the breast (Czank *et al.*, 2007).

Key fact

If the infant is incorrectly attached to the breast or unable to remove the breastmilk from the breast, there will be a build up of FIL culminating in a reduced supply of breastmilk. This can be rectified by regular and effective emptying of the breast by correcting positioning and attachment or expressing breastmilk at regular intervals. See Chapter 3 for further information.

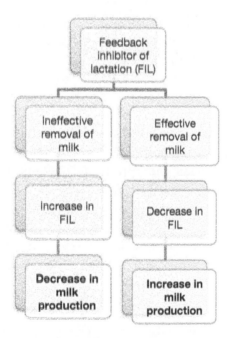

FIGURE 2.7 The autocrine/local response

> ## Practice recommendations
>
> - Ensure correct positioning and attachment at the breast to ensure effective removal of milk from the breast (see Chapter 3).
> - Promote baby-led feeding.
> - Avoid supplementary feeds such as formula milk and water, as this will lead to irregular removal of milk and subsequent build-up of FIL and a decrease in milk supply.
> - Increased stimulation of the breast through infant sucking or expression can lead to increased growth of secretory breast tissue and also induce lactation in non-lactating women.

Constituents of breastmilk

Types and properties of breastmilk

Colostrum

Colostrum is produced from approximately the sixteenth week of pregnancy (lactogenesis I) and is present and ready for birth. It develops into mature breastmilk around three to four days following the birth. Colostrum is a thick yellow/orange fluid that is a high-density but low-volume feed present in the first few days following birth, making it the ideal food for newborns. The small volumes facilitate the coordination of sucking, swallowing and breathing at the same time in the first few days of life. Newborns have immature kidneys and are only able to deal with small fluid volumes. Colostrum also has a purgative effect that helps clear the bowel of meconium, which has a high concentration of bile; this, in turn, reduces the possibility of jaundice (Lawrence and Lawrence, 2005).

Colostrum contains higher concentrations of antibodies, and anti-infective properties, such as IgA, lysosomes, lactoferrin and white blood cells, than mature milk. It is rich in growth factors and fat-soluble vitamins, particularly vitamin A (Stables and Rankin, 2010).

Transitional milk

This is the breastmilk produced in the first couple of weeks (lactogenesis II) in which the volume of milk gradually increases, the concentration of immunoglobins decreases and there is an increase in the calorific content, fat and lactose (Stables and Rankin, 2010).

Mature milk

The content of mature milk can vary between feeds. At the beginning of the feed it is high in protein, lactose and water – *'foremilk'*, and as the feed progresses the fat level gradually increases as the milk volume decreases – *'hindmilk'*. This is of particular importance when teaching mothers about the normal pattern of feeding (see Chapter 3). There is a significant increase in the fat content in the morning and early afternoon (Kent *et al.*, 2006).

Cregan *et al.* (2002) found the mean milk production for infants up to six months old over a 24-hour period was 809 ± 171ml, with a range between 549 and 1147ml, the highest volumes being removed in the morning. Kent (2007) suggested that the maternal energy requirement to produce an average of 759ml breastmilk per day is 630kcal.

Key fact

Some mothers worry about the appearance of the 'foremilk', believing it to lack substance because it is bluish in colour in the early feed, and will need reassurance that this is due to the lack of fat at the beginning of the feed.

The constituents of breastmilk

Breastmilk has many properties that meet the individual infant's needs and which, despite improvements in technology, cannot be accurately replicated in artificial milk; breastmilk is often referred to as a 'living fluid'. It is comprised of water, fat, protein, carbohydrates, electrolytes, minerals and immunoglobulins.

Key fact

Water makes up approximately 80 per cent of the milk volume and therefore infants do not need supplementary drinks, even in hot conditions.

Fat

This is the main source of energy and provides approximately half of the milk's calories. The lipids are mainly made up of globules of triglycerides, which are easy to digest and which make up 98 per cent of the fat content of breastmilk (RCM, 2009). Breastmilk contains long chain fatty acids, which aid brain and eye development, as well as the nervous and vascular system. However, fat content in breastmilk varies throughout a feed, increasing as the breast is emptied (Czank *et al.*, 2007). Full breasts are associated with minimum fat content of the milk, while emptier breasts are associated with higher fat content (Kent, 2007).

Protein

Mature breastmilk contains approximately 40 per cent casein and 60 per cent whey proteins, which form soft curds in the stomach and are easy to digest (Lawrence and Lawrence, 2005). The whey proteins contain anti-infective proteins, while casein is important to carry calcium and phosphate. *Lactoferrin* binds iron, promoting easier absorption and preventing the growth of bacteria in the intestine. *Bifidus factor* is also available to promote the growth of *lactobacillus bifidus* (good bacteria), to inhibit harmful bacteria by increasing the pH of the infant's stool. *Taurine* is also required for the conjugation of bile salts and absorption of fats in the first few days, as well as the myelination of the nervous system.

Prebiotics (oligosaccharides)

These interact with intestinal epithelial cells to stimulate the immune system, reduce gut pH to prevent pathogenic bacteria causing infection, and increase the numbers of bifido bacteria on the mucosa (Coppa *et al.*, 2004).

Carbohydrates

Lactose is the main carbohydrate in breastmilk (98 per cent) and can be quickly broken down into glucose. Lactose is important for brain growth and is found in higher concentration in human milk than in that of other mammals. Lactose is also important in the growth of lactobacillus bifidus. The amount of lactose in the breastmilk also regulates the volume of milk production through osmosis.

Iron

Breast-fed infants do not require iron supplements before the age of six months because the low levels of iron in breastmilk are bound by lactoferrin, making it more bio-available and thus preventing growth of bacteria in the intestine.

Artificial milk has approximately six times more 'free iron', which is less bio-available, thus promoting growth of bacteria and the risk of infection. Other trace elements are available in lower concentrations than in artificial milk but are considered ideal as they are readily absorbed (Walker, 2010).

Fat soluble vitamins

Concentrations of vitamin A and E are adequate for infants. However, vitamin D and K are not always at the desired level. Vitamin D is essential for bone development, but levels are dependent upon the mother's exposure to sunlight. The DH (SACN, 2007b) recommends that breastfeeding mothers take 10μg vitamin D supplements daily (see Chapter 7 for further details). Vitamin K is required for blood clotting. Colostrum has low levels of vitamin K and therefore vitamin K is administered routinely to infants at birth. As lactation matures and the infant's gut is colonised with bacteria, vitamin K levels rise (RCM, 2009).

Electrolytes and minerals

There is a third less electrolyte content in breastmilk compared to artificial milk and 0.2 per cent of sodium, potassium and chloride. Calcium, phosphorus and magnesium are present in breastmilk at higher concentrations than in plasma.

Immunoglobins

Immunoglobins are present in breastmilk in three ways and cannot be replicated in formula milk:

- antibodies from previous maternal infections;
- sIgA (secretory immunoglobin A), which lines the digestive tract;
- the entero-mammary and broncho-mammary pathways (gut-associated lymphatic tissue (GALT) and bronchus-associated lymphatic tissue (BALT). These detect infection in the mother's gastric or respiratory tract and produce antibodies.

White blood cells are present and act as a defensive mechanism to infection; viral fragments prime the baby's immune systems and anti-inflammatory molecules are thought to protect against necrotising enterocolitis by reducing inflammation in response to pathogens in the gut (Lawrence and Lawrence, 2005; Hale and Hartmann, 2007; Walker, 2010).

The RCM (2009) produced a useful booklet, *Infant Feeding: A Resource for Health Care Professionals and Parents*, which provides a comprehensive overview of the constituents of breastmilk and formula milk, and the safe storage of expressed breastmilk.

Volumes of breastmilk

It is important not to try and equate the number and volume of breastfeeds with formula milk. However, many mothers express concern about the amount of milk they are providing for their infants. The following is a guide to average volumes of breastmilk taken during breastfeeding (Kent, 2007):

* At birth   up to 5ml breastmilk   first breastfeed
* Within 24 hours   7–123ml/day breastmilk   3–8 breastfeeds
* Between 2–6 days   395–868ml/day breastmilk   5–10 breastfeeds
* One month   395–868ml/day breastmilk   6–18 breastfeeds
* Six months   710–803ml/day breastmilk   6–18 breastfeeds.

It is interesting to note that each breast produces different amounts of milk. In seven out of ten mothers the right breast was found to be more productive (Kent, 2007). Kent (2007) suggests that infants only empty the breast at one or two feeds per day and, on average, only 67 per cent of the milk available is consumed at an average volume of 76ml per feed.

Neonatal adaptation to life

Adaptation to extrauterine life

During pregnancy the mother provides a constant supply of nutrients to the fetus via the placenta. At birth, once the umbilical cord stops pulsating or is cut, there is an abrupt end to the continuous maternal provision of nutrients and the newborn has to adapt to intermittent feeding, and the major source of fuel changes from glucose to fat, either from colostrum or neonatal stores.

At birth, infants mobilise stored glucose and fatty acids until a feeding pattern is established. It is normal for plasma glucose levels to decrease within the first two to three hours of life. This coincides with a decreased level of plasma insulin and an increase in plasma triglycerides, fatty acids and glycerol (Rasmussen, 2007). It is normal for healthy breastfed infants to have lower plasma glucose and higher ketones until lactogenesis II commences than formula-fed infants.

In the normal healthy term infant, blood glucose levels will drop to approximately 2.6mmol/l (WHO, 1977) or 2.0mmol/l (NICE, 2008b) (see local protocol) following birth, but gradually rise to approximately 3.6mmol/l after about six hours. In response to low plasma glucose, serum glucagon levels rise, converting intracellular glycogen stores to glucose (glycogenolysis). The high levels of glucose lead to increased levels of insulin and decreased glucagon levels, but the stores of glycogen will decrease rapidly over the first 24 hours after birth. The newborn also has the ability to mobilise alternative fuels through lipolysis and ketogenesis. This is a normal physiological process and therefore there is no reason to monitor blood glucose levels within the first two to four hours as it will only encourage unnecessary intervention.

Healthy term infants are born with glycogen and fat stores to meet their nutritional needs within the first few days of life while they learn to suckle and feed from the breast. As discussed earlier, colostrum provides all the nutrients required in the first few days of life. The small volume of colostrum, approximately 5ml at the first feed (Kent, 2007), encourages the coordination of sucking, breathing and swallowing. Due to the small volumes of colostrum, newborn infants will feed regularly and as a result blood glucose levels are maintained; there is early evacuation of meconium due to the purgative effect of colostrum (reducing the possibility of jaundice); there is promotion of the hormones of lactation, and the mother–baby bond is established.

The mechanisms of suckling

To enable effective removal of breastmilk, human infants are 'hardwired' to suck at birth; however, the birthing environment must support these natural mechanisms. Sucking movements have been observed in utero from 14 weeks, but it is not until 32 weeks' gestation that the fetus/premature infant is able to coordinate the suck and swallow responses, and approximately 34–36 weeks' gestation to suck, swallow, breathe and feed at the breast (UNICEF, 2008a).

Neurobehavioural programme

Nils Bergman (2008) described the transition to extrauterine life as the critical period of birth, suggesting there is a window of opportunity whereby the infant's innate survival programmes are developed or suppressed. He suggests a newborn's behaviour is directed by the limbic system via the autonomic nervous system, hormonal system and muscular (somatic) system. Together they achieve the optimum state for current and future health, development and well-being.

Bergman (2008) states that, at birth, an infant's senses are primed to receive new stimuli without filters. However, filters quickly develop as a learning response. Bergman identifies the mother's smell and skin-to-skin contact as the most important stimuli at birth, as this directly affects emotional memory and fear conditioning. He recommends filters, such as separation, be avoided at this time and that the mother–infant dyad be left undisturbed for a minimum of one hour. This should not be viewed as a one-off process; instead, mother–infant contact should be encouraged as an ongoing process where possible.

Bergman (2008) describes the interplay of the autonomic nervous system, hormonal system and muscular (somatic) system in the process of '*self-attachment*' in which infants, who have not been subject to filters, are observed crawling and attaching to the breast. Skin-to-skin contact at birth encourages the following neurobehavioural programme for suckling:

1 waking and stretching;
2 hand-to-mouth movements;
3 open mouth, tongue movement and licking;
4 crawling to the nipple;
5 massaging the breast;
6 attaching to the breast.

Crying is a late cue and can cause problems with attaching to the breast.

The prone position of skin-to-skin contact allows the infant to move its neck and lead with the chin to find the nipple (*rooting response*). When the infant reaches the nipple, it brushes against the philtrum (between nose and upper lip) and the infant opens its mouth in a 'wide gape' (*gape response*). It takes a mouthful of nipple and surrounding breast tissue and begins to suck. Matthiesen *et al.* (2001) video-recorded and observed ten newborn infants in skin-to-skin contact from birth to the first breastfeed; the mothers had not had analgesia. They found that the infants used their hands as well as mouths to stimulate the breasts, resulting in oxytocin release in a coordinated fashion.

Sucking

It was thought that newborn infants predominantly used 'tongue stripping', a wave-like motion, to strip milk from the breast (positive pressure). This peristaltic movement of the tongue moves from the anterior aspect of the mouth to the posterior and is in contrast to the up-and-down motion of the formula-fed infant. In 1986, Woolridge and Drewett described the role of both the positive pressure exerted by the milk-ejection reflex and the negative pressure in the infant's mouth where suction occurs due to the vacuum created in the mouth. In a more recent study using ultrasound to observe the movements of the tongue during breastfeeding, Geddes (2007b) found that vacuum (negative pressure) played a greater role in the removal of milk than previously thought, suggesting that the creation of negative pressure is an essential component of this process.

Geddes (2007b) described the nipple/areola being drawn into the mouth by negative pressure to the anterior point of the junction of the hard and soft palate. A teat is formed and the vacuum (–60mmHg) holds the teat in place. Vacuum occurs as the tongue and jaw move down, drawing milk from the breast. She suggests that the peristaltic movement of the tongue does not occur; instead, as the tongue rises, the vacuum decreases reducing milk flow.

At term, the design of the newborn's mouth assists with this action as the tongue is large, filling the mouth alongside the breast. The cheeks also have thick pads of fat and muscle, *buccinators*, which prevent collapse when the tongue depresses during sucking. If the cheeks collapse (appear drawn in) this reduces the negative pressure. The *temporalis* and *masseter* muscles coordinate the symmetrical movement of the jaw during sucking, raising the mandible during the positive pressure phase of the suck and lowering it during the negative pressure phase. The newborn is able to protect its airway from aspiration because the epiglottis and soft palate touch at rest, diverting the milk to the oesophagus (Genna, 2008).

During attachment to the breast the lower lip flanges outward on the breast. If the upper lip is also flanged out, this may be a sign of poor attachment. The muscle above the lips, *orbicularis oris*, contracts to maintain the seal and the *mentalis muscle* at the lower lip assists feeding by elevating and protruding the lower lip (Genna, 2008).

Swallowing

Coordinated swallowing is evident from 32–34 weeks' gestation. It is triggered by the bolus of milk that accumulates between the palate and the tongue. Genna (2008, pp. 10–12) describes four phases to sucking:

1   *Oral preparatory phase*: This involves rooting, attachment and sucking. As the jaw drops negative pressure is exerted, creating a vacuum to encourage milk to flow from the breast. The tongue forms a trough to channel the milk to the back of the mouth.
2   *Oral transitory phase*: Milk is propelled to the back of the mouth.
3   *Pharyngeal phase*: This involves airway protection. Breathing stops, the soft palate rises to close off the nasal cavity, the vocal cords close the trachea and the hyoid bones rise anteriorly, elevating the larynx. As the tongue

moves posteriorly, the vacuum reduces and milk flow ceases, the epiglottis moves back and downwards, closing the larynx and diverting the milk bolus to the oesophagus. This is assisted by the contraction of the pharyngeal wall and opening of the oesophageal sphincter.

4 *Oesophageal phase*: The milk bolus passes through the oesophagus aided by peristaltic movement.

However, up-and-down jaw movements are not defining characteristics of good attachment and swallowing. Walker (2010, p. 151) suggests that the following are good signs of swallowing:

* deep jaw movement;
* audible sounds of swallowing;
* vibration on the occipital area of the head (felt by hand).

Breathing

As breathing must be coordinated with sucking and swallowing, the airway must be protected. An extended neck assists stabilisation of the airway and, in contrast, flexion of the neck increases the risk of collapse of the airway.

Concluding comments

There appears to be a plethora of new research about breastfeeding in recent years from anatomy and physiology to the mechanism of suckling and infant behaviour. To be able to advise and adequately support mothers with breastfeeding, it is crucial that healthcare professionals keep up to date with research and develop a good understanding of how breastfeeding works, in order to underpin their practice and to be able to effectively pass this information on to mothers in language they understand. The following chapter will explore the essential skills required for practice.

True or false quiz

		True	or False
1	The size of the lactating breast is determined by glandular tissue.	☐	☐
2	All mothers produce a similar amount of breastmilk.	☐	☐
3	Lactiferous ducts can be found 5–8mm from the nipple.	☐	☐
4	Mothers have one milk ejection during a breastfeed.	☐	☐
5	Some breastfed infants may need water between feeds.	☐	☐
6	Colostrum has a purgative effect on the infant bowel.	☐	☐
7	The fat content of breastmilk is higher at the end of the feed.	☐	☐
8	The factors present in breastmilk that protect the infant from infection are replicated in formula milk.	☐	☐
9	Prolactin is inhibited until the third stage of labour is complete.	☐	☐
10	A build-up of the feedback inhibitor of lactation will increase milk production.	☐	☐

Further reading

- Geddes, D. (2007) 'Inside the lactating breast: the latest anatomy research', *Journal of Midwifery and Women's Health*, 52(6): 556–63.
- Genna, C.W. (2008) *Supporting Sucking Skills in Breastfeeding*, London: Jones and Bartlett.
- Hale, T. and Hartmann, P. (eds) (2007) *Textbook of Human Lactation*, Amarillo, TX: Hale Publishing.
- Hilton, S. (2008) 'Milk production during pregnancy and beyond', *British Journal of Midwifery*, 16(8): 544–8.
- Royal College of Midwifery (RCM) (2009) *Infant Feeding: A Resource for Health Care Professionals and Parents*. London: RCM Trust.

Chapter 3 **Essential skills for practice**

- Learning outcomes
- Teaching positioning and attachment
- Assessing a breastfeed
- Expressing breastmilk
- Storage of expressed breastmilk
- Concluding comments
- Quiz
- Resources

The *Infant Feeding Survey 2005* (Bolling *et al.*, 2007) reported that nine out of ten mothers gave up breastfeeding before they had wanted to, only seven in ten were shown how to put their infant to the breast in the first few days, and a third of mothers experienced problems in hospital or within the first few weeks. Healthcare professionals' lack of knowledge and skills to support mothers to breastfeed their infants have been identified as a major contributing factor to low rates of initiation and duration of breastfeeding, leading to inconsistent and inaccurate advice (Renfrew *et al.*, 2005). This chapter focuses on the essential skills required to effectively support breastfeeding, such as effective positioning and attachment, assessing a breastfeed, hand expression, the use of pumps and, finally, storage of milk.

Learning outcomes

By the end of this chapter you will be able to:

- demonstrate effective positioning and attachment of an infant at the breast;
- observe and assess a complete breastfeed;
- teach a mother how to hand express her breastmilk and safely store it;
- describe the safe and effective use of breast pumps.

Mapping the UNICEF UK BFI educational outcomes

2   Have developed an in-depth knowledge of the physiology of lactation and be able to apply this in practical situations.

3   Be able to recognise effective positioning, attachment and suckling and to empower mothers to develop the skills necessary for them to achieve these for themselves.

4   Be able to demonstrate knowledge of the principles of hand expression and have the ability to teach these to mothers.

8   Be equipped to provide parents with accurate, evidence-based information about activities which may have an impact on breastfeeding.

Teaching positioning and attachment

Positions for breastfeeding

It is important that breastfeeding mothers understand the need for a comfortable and sustainable position when establishing breastfeeding, in order to avoid poor attachment at the breast that will result in ineffective removal of the milk and trauma. Good positioning is different for each mother as many variables are present, such as the size of the breasts. However, there are some principles that mothers should be taught to help them achieve a good position for effective and sustained attachment at the breast (UNICEF, 2008a):

- ✔ *The mother should adopt a position she can sustain.* If she is not comfortable this may cut the breastfeed short and the infant will not benefit from the full-fat milk at the end of the feed. It will also encourage a build-up of FIL and consequently reduce the milk supply.
- ✔ *Head and neck should be in a straight line.* This enables the infant to open its mouth wide, with the tongue on the base of the mouth to scoop up the

breast. Avoid twisting of the head and neck as this also helps protect the airway and encourages a successful suck-swallow-breathe reflex.

✔ *Allow the infant to move its head freely*. Avoiding holding the back of the infant's head is critical for successful breastfeeding; instead, the infant's neck and shoulders should be supported so that it can freely move its head to find the correct position to lead with the chin, keep the nose free and open the mouth with a wide gape. It also allows the infant to extend its neck and stabilise its airway during the suck-swallow-breathe reflex. In contrast, holding the head pushes the nose, top lip and mouth to the breast, flexing the neck. This will cause obstruction of the airway and may block the nose against the breast. It may also encourage the mother to press her breast with her fingers to produce a gap to allow the infant to breathe and, in doing so, prevent milk flow and interfere with attachment. By allowing the infant the freedom to extend the neck, it encourages it to approach the breast chin first to scoop the breast into the mouth and keep the nostrils free. Pushing the head against the breast may also result in breast refusal.

✔ *Hold the infant close*. Bring the infant to the breast rather than the breast to the infant, as this would distort the shape of the breast.

✔ *Nose should be to nipple*. This encourages the infant to tilt its head backwards and lead with the chin. In this position the tongue will also remain at the base of the mouth so that the nipple is aimed at the junction of the hard and soft palate.

✔ *Approach the breast chin first*. The chin will indent the breast, the lower lip will flange outwards and the infant will scoop the breast into the mouth (see Figure 3.2 on page 50).

In the early days of breastfeeding, a mother will require support to find comfortable positions. Advise her to make sure that her clothing is not restricting the feed or that hair or jewellery are not in the way. Many mothers feel thirsty when breastfeeding, so having a drink at hand is a good idea. Usually mothers can sustain positions where they feel supported by furniture or pillows. Each mother will need to be assessed individually. Considering pillows to support her back or a footstool if required may be helpful. If she has a painful perineum she may need a cushion to sit on. When lying flat, using pillows to support her back or head may make the position more comfortable. It may be useful for mothers of small infants to place them on a pillow on the mother's lap; this will depend on the size and shape of the mother's breast because this can be a hindrance to larger infants or mothers with large breasts, causing the infant to assume a twisted position.

Some mothers may need additional help and assistance in the early days, particularly if they have not breastfed before. In some hospitals as many as one in three or four mothers will have had a Caesarean section. They will need advice on the best positions to avoid the infant lying on the Caesarean section wound. Mothers of twins will need additional help to position the infants. These mothers are at greater risk of shorter duration of breastfeeding (Baxter, 2006) (see Chapter 6 for further discussion).

Some mothers find it helpful to support their breasts, particularly if they are soft or large. This can be done by placing the fingers flat against the ribs, under the breast, with the thumb at a right angle to the fingers. Mothers should be advised to avoid shaping the breast as this may inhibit the flow of breastmilk and potentially cause trauma. As long as the principles above are adhered to, the infant can feed in any position in a 360° circumference of the breast. The following are examples of the more common positions mothers use (see Figure 3.1).

- *The cradle position* is the most common position, where the mother sits upright and the infant's neck and shoulders are supported by the mother's forearm or bend in the elbow. Care must be taken not to restrict movement of the head.
- *The cross-cradle position* is similar except that the baby is supported by the forearm and the neck and shoulders by the mother's hand. It is important that the infant's head is free to move to attain optimal attachment on the breast.
- *The underarm hold* is suitable particularly following a Caesarean section to avoid pressure on the wound. Again the mother sits upright and she holds the infant to the side, tucking the infant's trunk under her arm with its feet towards her back.
- *Lying down/on the side* is particularly useful if the mother is tired or has a sore perineum. The infant faces the breast, body in alignment, nose to nipple.
- *Straddling* the infant over the mother's legs with the infant sat upright facing the breast is helpful if the infant has congenital hip dislocation.
- *Leaning over the baby* can be useful if the mother has a blocked duct and wants to change the angle of the feed. She places the infant on a secure flat surface, leans over the infant and allows it to attach to the breast as usual. This is also useful for mothers with inverted nipples as the gravity helps the infant to take a mouthful of breast.

Attachment to the breast

The infant's rooting and suckling reflexes will be stimulated by gentle tactile stimulation of the breast. Once the infant has turned towards the nipple and

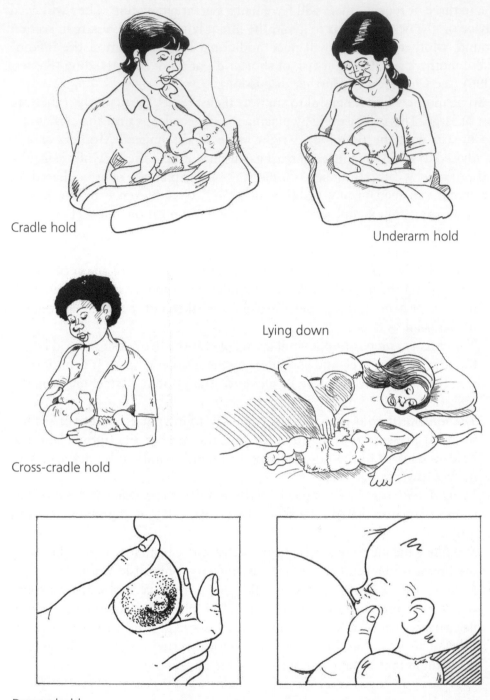

Cradle hold

Underarm hold

Lying down

Cross-cradle hold

Dancer hold

FIGURE 3.1 Positions for breastfeeding

Source: adapted from © UNICEF UK BFI.

touched it with its lower lip, the reflex to open its mouth will be stimulated (Both and Frischknect, 2008). The infant will open its mouth wide, with the tongue to the base of the mouth. If the mouth is not open wide enough, or the tongue is in the roof of the mouth, the infant will be unable to attach effectively to the breast, resulting in 'nipple sucking' and consequently sore nipples and ineffective milk removal, which may result in insufficient milk supply. Poor attachment can be the precursor to a number of problems that will be discussed in greater detail throughout this book.

The mother must be taught the signs of correct attachment to ensure successful breastfeeding, which are (UNICEF, 2008a):

✔ wide-open mouth, tongue on the base of the mouth, scooping a large mouthful of breast;
✔ chin indenting the breast;
✔ lower lip curled out and upper lip in a neutral position;
✔ full cheeks;
✔ the sound of swallowing;
✔ seeing milk at the sides of the mouth;
✔ more areola visible above the top lip than the bottom (although difficult for the mother to see in a sitting position).

Effective attachment (see Figure 3.2) is crucial for successful breastfeeding and midwives and health visitors must develop the skills to assess and advise mothers. This is particularly the case in a bottle-feeding culture, where many mothers may not have witnessed successful breastfeeding before and there is a lack of support from family and friends. However, in a minority of mothers, there may be particular challenges that make it difficult for the infant to attach to the breast. These will be explored further in Chapters 5, 6 and 7.

Ineffective attachment

Poor attachment at the breast can lead to a plethora of problems for the mother and infant. For the mother, poor attachment may lead to sore or cracked nipples. If the infant is not properly attached to the breast this will result in ineffective removal and stasis of breastmilk, leading to engorgement, blocked ducts, mastitis and possible abscess (UNICEF, 2008a). Because there is ineffective removal of breastmilk there will be a build-up of the FIL, resulting in a reduced production of breastmilk. The shape of the lactocytes will be distorted, preventing prolactin binding to it and thus slowing down and ultimately preventing further milk production (Czank et al., 2007).

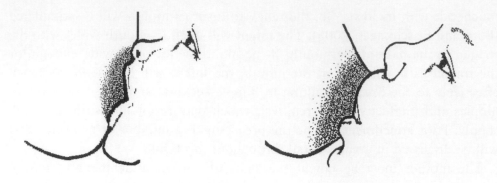

Effective attachment at the breast   Ineffective attachment at the breast

FIGURE 3.2 Attachment at the breast

Source: © UNICEF UK BFI.

A poor milk supply will lead to the infant becoming unsatisfied, feeding for a long time or becoming frustrated, reluctance to go to the breast and being difficult to settle. The infant is unlikely to empty the breast sufficiently to receive the fattier milk as the breast empties and will become colicky and have explosive, watery and frothy stools. Ultimately, this will lead to poor weight gain and failure to thrive (UNICEF, 2008a). Many mothers perceive this as an inability to produce enough milk to satisfy their infant rather than a problem with technique.

Feeding pattern

At the beginning of a feed before milk ejection, the sucking bursts are rapid, shallow and long with infrequent pauses to swallow. If this continues it can be a sign of poor milk transfer (Watson-Genna and Sandora, 2008). As the feed progresses the bursts become slower and shorter, and the pauses longer, until the end of the feed when sucks become like flutters and the infant releases the breast. The end of the feed is extremely important and the mother should be informed not to take the infant off the breast prematurely but, instead, to wait for the infant to release the breast itself, because the fat content of the breastmilk is at its highest at that point (see Figure 3.3). A sign of good attachment is that the nipple should have maintained a round shape and not be distorted (UNICEF, 2008a). It is difficult to give a time limit for the length of feeds as this is individual to each infant. At the end of the feed the infant will become more relaxed and will let go of the breast; the nipple should look round and healthy. In the first few weeks it is normal for infants to feed approximately 8–12 times a day.

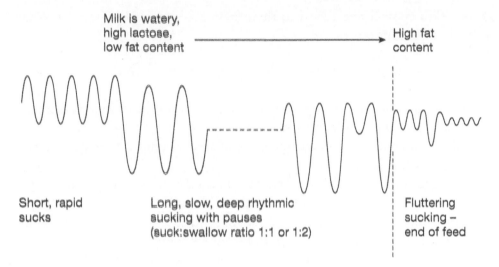

FIGURE 3.3 The feeding pattern

It is important that healthcare professionals recognise factors that affect infants' feeding behaviour. To do this they must have knowledge and understanding of oral and feeding development in the fetus and newborn (see Chapter 2). Gestational age, illnesses and separation of the mother–infant dyad will undoubtedly have an effect and will be discussed further in Chapter 7. Maternal factors such as common problems, medication and medical conditions will also be considered in Chapters 4, 5 and 6.

Signs of ineffective attachment in the feeding pattern

- If the infant continues with rapid sucks and does not demonstrate signs of slow rhythmic sucking, this can be a sign of poor attachment.
- Very long feeds and frequent feeds/very short feeds.
- Colic and frothy, watery stool.
- Breast refusal (UNICEF, 2008a).

See Chapter 5 for the management of the consequences of incorrect attachment.

Biological nurturing

Suzanne Colson (2010) defines biological nurturing as 'any mother/infant behaviour at the breast where the infant is in close chest contact with the mother's body contours'. Ultimately, biological nurturing offers unrestricted

skin-to-skin contact and access to the breast. Colson (2010) states biological nurturing assumptions as:

- Mothers and infants are versatile feeders. There is not one way to breast-feed.
- A baby does not need to be awake to latch on and feed. Infants often self-attach; mothers can help them do this.
- Infants often have reflex movements called 'cues', indicating they are ready to feed while asleep.
- Looking for baby reflex feeding cues helps mothers to get to know their infants sooner. This increases confidence.
- Crying and hunger cues are late feeding indicators often making latching difficult. Getting started with breastfeeding is about releasing infant feeding reflexes as stimulants, helping infants find the breast, latch on and feed . . . not about interest.
- The breastfeeding position the baby uses often mimics that in the womb.
- There is no right or wrong breastfeeding position. The right position is the one that works.
- Infants do not always feed for hunger; 'non-nutritive sucking' is hugely beneficial to increase your milk and satisfy your baby's needs.

However, some healthcare professionals are concerned that Colson's methods are in conflict with the BFI initiative. In November 2008, the BFI invited Suzanne Colson to speak at their conference. This was followed in February 2009 by a statement on their website in response to questions from professionals as to whether they should replace the skills recommended in Step 5 of the *Ten Steps* and Point 4 of the *Seven Point Plan*. The BFI states that they do not oppose Dr Colson's methods and acknowledge that biological nurturing is of benefit in the early postpartum period, particularly where there are attachment problems and breast refusal, and that it reinforces the benefits of skin-to-skin contact. However, the BFI advises caution about replacing the current methods of teaching positioning and attachment, highlighting the point that mothers need to be equipped with the basic information about how breastfeeding works and how to position their infants correctly to the breast in a variety of situations where biological nurturing may not be possible in order to avoid problems.

For further information on biological nurturing see www.biological nurturing.com.

Assessing a breastfeed

There are several tools available to help healthcare professionals to assess breastfeeding technique and to make recommendations for changes to improve breastfeeding outcome. The BFI recommends that a breastfeeding assessment be carried out on day five, including assessment of milk transfer (UNICEF, 2010e). It developed a checklist to help healthcare professionals observe breastfeeding before, during and after a feed (see Table 3.1). However, there are other indicators that breastfeeding and the transfer of milk is successful, such as observing nappies for urine output and stool, and weight gain.

Assessing urine and stool

Urine and stool output are fundamental indicators that an infant is feeding well and can be easily recognised by the parents if they are taught to do so. Researchers in California (Nommsen-Rivers *et al.*, 2008) believe that in order for women to assess their own breastfeeding they need to be able to assess wet and soiled nappies. They asked 242 mothers to rate the soiled nappies and fullness of their breasts. They found the most effective sign of poor breastfeeding was on day four if there were three or fewer soiled (with stool) nappies. Urine output was less accurate as the mothers were less able to identify this in the nappy. By day three the infant would be expected to produce at least three wet nappies in 24 hours and from day five to six, six or more wet nappies (see Table 3.2).

The first stool is meconium, which is thick black/green and tarry. This will change over the first few days and is called the 'changing stool' or 'transitional stool'. If the infant is feeding well the stool can be expected to be yellow by day four or five (see Table 3.2).

During the first six weeks it would be expected that a breastfed infant would produce frequent stools ($\geqslant 2$ per day). Older infants may have gaps of several days.

Urates and pseudo-menstruation

Urates, which look like orange/pinkish crystals, may be found in the nappy. Parents should be informed that they are salts in the urine and be reassured this is normal for some infants in the first few days. However, urates can be a sign that the infant needs to feed more often or more effectively. This may be a good time to reassess positioning and attachment to prevent any further problems.

TABLE 3.1 UNICEF UK BFI Breastfeeding Observation Checklist

Signs that breastfeeding is going well	*Signs of possible difficulty*

Before attachment:

Mother's position

__ Mother relaxed and comfortable	__ Mother not relaxed, e.g. shoulders tense
__ Breast hanging or lying naturally[1]	__ Breast squashed or restricted
__ Easy access to nipple/areola	__ Access to nipple/areola restricted
__ Hair/clothing do not restrict mother's view	__ Mother's view restricted by hair/clothing

Baby's position

__ Baby's head and body in line	__ Baby has to twist head and neck to feed
__ Baby held close to mother's body	__ Baby not held close to mother's body
__ [Baby's whole body supported][2]	__ [Only shoulders or head supported]
__ Baby's nose opposite nipple	__ Baby's lower lip/chin opposite nipple

Attaching to the breast:

__ Baby reaches or roots for the breast	__ No response to the breast
__ Mother waits for baby to open mouth wide	__ Mother does not wait for baby to 'gape'
__ Baby opens mouth wide	__ Baby does not open mouth wide
__ Mother brings baby swiftly towards breast	__ Mother does not move baby in swiftly
__ Baby's chin/lower lip/tongue touches breast first	__ Baby's top lip touches the breast first

During the feed:

Observations

__ Baby's chin touches the breast	__ Baby's chin does not touch the breast
__ Baby's mouth wide open	__ Baby's mouth pursed, lips point forward
__ Baby's cheeks soft and rounded	__ Baby's cheeks tense or pulled in
__ Baby's lower lip turned outwards	__ Baby's lower lip turned in
__ If visible, more areola above baby's top lip[3]	__ More areola seen below bottom lip (or equal)
__ Breasts remain round during a feed	__ Breasts look stretched or pulled
__ Signs of milk release (e.g. leaking)	__ No signs of milk release

Baby's behaviour

__ Baby stays attached to the breast	__ Baby slips off the breast
__ Baby calm and alert at the breast	__ Baby restless or fussy
__ Slow, deep sucking bursts with pauses	__ Rapid shallow sucks
__ No noise other than swallowing	__ Smacking or clicking sounds
__ Rhythmic swallowing seen	__ Occasional or no swallowing seen

At the end of the feed:

__ Baby releases the breast spontaneously	__ Mother takes baby off the breast
__ Breasts appear soft	__ Breasts are hard or inflamed
__ Nipple is same shape as before feed	__ Nipple is wedge-shaped or squashed
__ Skin of nipple/areola appears healthy	__ Nipple/areola is sore or cracked

Source: UNICEF (2008a, p. 74).

1 If the mother prefers her breast to be supported, this should not move it from its natural lie.
2 The observations in square brackets [ ] are less important in older babies than in the newborn.
3 This may not be significant if the mother's nipple is not in the centre of her areola.

TABLE 3.2 Assessing a nappy

Day	Wet nappies per day	Stools per day
1–2	Two or more	One (meconium – green/black and sticky)
3–4	Three or more (getting heavier)	Three or more (changing stool)
4–6	Five or more (heavy, approx. 45ml)	Three or more (yellow)
Up to six weeks	Six or more (heavy)	At least two (yellow, 'seedy' in appearance)

Another concern parents may have is pseudo-menstruation. This is a very light bleed from the vagina in some girls and is a result of oestrogen withdrawal. Parents should be reassured that this is normal.

Weighing

All infants are expected to lose weight within the first few days of life, which is thought to be due to normal fluid loss. At birth infants are born with extra interstitial fluid in their tissues which needs to be reduced. Approximately 80 per cent of infants regain their birthweight within two weeks of age and less than 5 per cent lose greater than 10 per cent (DH, 2009c). A normal weight loss is currently considered to be up to 7 per cent of the birthweight, after which the minimum weight gain should be 20g per day, and by day 14 the infant should have regained the birthweight.

A weight loss of between 7 and 12 per cent of the birthweight is indicative that the infant is not getting enough milk. A weight loss of above 12 per cent should be referred to either the general practitioner (GP) or paediatrician.

Weight loss must be calculated as a percentage using the following formula:

$$\frac{\text{weight loss (g)}}{\text{birthweight (g)}} \times 100 = \text{weight loss (\%)}$$

Therefore, if the birthweight is 3800g, the weight loss will be:

$$\frac{200\text{g}}{3800\text{g}} \times 100 = 5.2\%.$$

In 2009, the WHO introduced 0–4 years growth charts for all new births. These charts are based on the growth of breastfed infants. The WHO found that infants worldwide had similar growth patterns and developed the new

---

Activity

Read your local guidelines for routine infant weighing policy. The usual pattern for weighing infants initially is at birth (including home births); between days four and six (usually when the blood spot test is done); and around day 10 or 11.

---

chart based on data from children who exclusively breastfed for a minimum of four months and partially for one year. The data were collected from infants with no health or environmental factors that may impair the normal growth pattern (DH, 2009c). The new charts include a separate preterm section for infants 32–36 weeks' gestation; a chart for preterm infants born before 32 weeks' gestation; no centile lines between 0–2 weeks; and the fiftieth centile has been de-emphasised (DH, 2009c, p. 5). The DH recommends that all users of the new growth charts undertake training.

Materials for training can be downloaded from www.growthcharts. rcph.ac.uk. Guidelines are also available on the Department of Health's website, www.dh.gov.uk/publications.

The DH recommends class III electronic scales in the metric setting for weighing children up to the age of two years, removing all clothing. All weighing equipment must be in good working order and regularly maintained. The same equipment should be used where possible to avoid any error and all staff should be trained in the use of the equipment and implications of the findings.

Expressing breastmilk

Hand expression

Hand expression is a fundamental technique that should be taught to a mother within 24 hours following birth so that she is confident to deal with any issues that may arise, such as supplementing a breastfeed if the infant is ill, or unable to breastfeed well at the breast, or if they are separated for any reason. It also helps her resolve other challenges such as inverted nipples or engorgement. Hand expression is recommended rather than a breast pump because, in the first few days, colostrum levels are low and may get lost in a breast pump apparatus (UNICEF, 2008a). Hand expression also provides tactile stimulus, which encourages the hormones of lactation and enables the mother to target specific sites in the breast if she has blocked ducts. If hand expression is the only means of emptying the breast, the mother should be encouraged to express breastmilk at least eight times a day, including during the night when prolactin levels are highest (UNICEF, 2010e).

The BFI (UNICEF, 2008a, p. 31) suggests that teaching mothers the correct technique for hand expression, as well as a rationale for how breastfeeding works, gives mothers confidence and empowers them to deal with challenges if they arise. Teaching hand expression is best done using a breast model. A 'hands off' approach should be used unless the mother requests otherwise. There are also leaflets that can be given to the mother that describe the procedure in words and pictures; these can be useful teaching aids (see DH and UNICEF UK BFI websites).

Good breast massage is essential to stimulate milk ejection and should be performed prior to hand expression or when using a pump (Jones and Spencer, 2008). Any of the following techniques can be used; it depends which the mother finds most comfortable and acceptable:

- Stroke the breast with gentle feather-like movement or gently roll knuckles from the top of the breast towards the areola.
- Roll the nipple between the thumb and forefinger.
- Stroke under the nipple and areola with the palm of the hand in an upward movement.

Other ways to assist milk ejection are to express near the infant if possible or have a photograph or a piece of the infant's clothing nearby; the smells and sounds of the infant stimulate milk ejection – the let-down. Anxiety is a known inhibitor of the let-down reflex (Lawrence and Lawrence, 2005) and therefore consideration must be given to the environment, particularly if it is not the mother's own home. In the hospital a private area should be offered where she knows she will not be interrupted. Physical comfort is also important and therefore the mother should be reminded to empty her bladder before commencing, and ensure she has a comfortable chair, a drink nearby and anything else she may need.

Teaching hand expression

- Wash hands with soap and water but not the breast before expressing. Good daily hygiene is sufficient.
- Have a clean container to collect the breastmilk and a towel to place under the breast in case of spillage.
- Encourage the mother to feel gently around the area of the areola where she will feel a different consistency in the tissue.

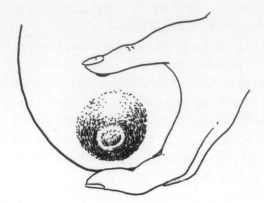

1. Thumb and first finger in a 'C' shape at 6 and 12 o'clock, approximately 2–3cms above nipple

2. Gently compress and release to express the breastmilk

FIGURE **3.4** Hand expression

- Ask her to place her thumb and first two fingers in a 'C' shape, at 6 and 12 o'clock, approximately 2–3cms above the nipple.
- She should then gently compress the breast and release to express the breastmilk. Some mothers may need to compress the breast and push back to the chest wall. Mothers will find their own rhythm.
- As the drops of breastmilk reduce and stop, she should move her fingers to a different position to drain all the ducts. However, this will not be necessary if the purpose of the expression is just to soften the breast.
- Mothers should be taught to avoid squeezing or sliding their fingers over the skin as this may cause breast tissue damage. They should also avoid pulling on the nipple as this may cause trauma.

It is important to remind mothers that, in the first few days following birth, volumes of colostrum are low and not to expect too much. Once they gain confidence some mothers may choose to hand express both breasts at the same time.

Breast pumps

Mothers are increasingly using breast pumps as part of their breastfeeding 'toolkit' and it is therefore imperative that healthcare professionals can support and advise them on the benefits and risks of their use and also how to use them safely. Mothers of preterm infants use them to establish and maintain milk supply. Others use breast pumps to express breastmilk for when they are separated from the infant for an evening out or to return to work. However, if used incorrectly, breast pumps can cause pain, nipple and breast tissue damage, milk contamination and infection (Buckley, 2009). Buckley (2009) described the breast pump as a 'double-edged sword'; on one side it is invaluable for mothers and infants with breastfeeding problems, but on the other side there are risks. She questions whether healthcare professionals recommend the use of breast pumps too quickly rather than using clinical observation, teaching the skill of hand expression and providing adequate support and advice.

Electronic breast pumps are comprised of a breast shield that sits over the nipple and areola on the breast and the pump, which creates the vacuum to express the milk. They are designed to imitate the infant's suckling, vacuum and sucking rhythm; 2-phase pumps begin with a faster rhythm, to initiate the let-down reflex, gradually slowing down as the milk flows. Equipment can be bought or rented. It is helpful if midwives and health visitors can provide a list of local organisations that provide a rental service. Some mothers buy hand pumps, which are cheaper and can be either electronic or manually operated. Suction is created by pumping a handle, but it can be very tiring.

Activity

Write a list of suppliers in your local area where mothers can either buy or rent breast pumps with single-use kits.

If the mother is using a pump to express milk to provide or supplement the infant's nutritional needs, the same instructions regarding how often to do this must be given as for hand expression (see 'Hand expression' above).

Not all breast shields fit all mothers and care must be taken to ensure the shield fits well and will not cause tissue damage. If the procedure is painful the breast shield could be either too big or too small. Different sizes are available from the manufacturer.

Double pumping (both breasts at the same time) is a good option for mothers who are expressing regularly, as it saves time and increases prolactin levels and therefore milk production. For single pumping the session should last approximately 15 minutes at each breast, but with double pumping it should be 10–15 minutes in total.

The mother should:

- prepare the environment to reduce anxiety levels and aid comfort, and have a memoir of the baby if it is not possible to express near the infant;
- wash hands with soap and water; and use a clean pump set (single-person use in hospital);
- use breast massage to encourage the let-down reflex and continue throughout the procedure;
- find a comfortable position that can be maintained;
- support the breast with the fingers flat against the ribs, under the breast and with the thumb at a right angle to the fingers;
- ensure the nipple is placed in the centre of the funnel of the breast shield; the mother should not press the funnel too hard against the breast tissue as this will cause trauma; however, she should make sure it is close enough to maintain the vacuum;
- start the vacuum on minimum and gradually increase; Kent *et al.* (2008) found in a small study of 23 mothers that expressing breastmilk at a mother's maximum comfortable vacuum enhanced milk flow and yield;
- not remove the shield while the vacuum is still on as this will cause nipple or breast trauma.

Kent *et al.* (2008) recommend that mothers use the maximum comfortable vacuum of a breast pump to maximise milk flow rate and yield. At this level they found there was an average of 4.3 milk ejections in a 15-minute period of expression, yielding 118.5ml of breastmilk, which is approximately 65 per cent of the available milk.

Mothers should be advised not to reduce the amount of pumping if the milk yield increases beyond what is needed by the infant, because if milk is only collected from the first phase of pumping it will not contain the high fat content of the later milk production. Also, if the intervals between pumping increase, this will lead to a decreased milk production due to the build up of FIL and reduced prolactin. Instead, the excess could be frozen or offered as donor milk (see Chapter 8 for donor milk guidelines).

Cleaning breast pump equipment

Each set of breast pump equipment must be used by one individual only, never shared even after cleaning. Single-person use equipment must also be thoroughly cleaned after each use. There is some debate about methods of sterilising equipment, but many areas are moving towards thorough washing, rinsing and dry storage (Gilks *et al.*, 2008) (review your local policy).

- Wash hands and ensure all surfaces are clean.
- Wash breast pump sets in hot soapy water. Ensure all milk is removed from all components. At home they can be cleaned in the dishwasher.
- Dry thoroughly with paper towels. At home they can be left to dry upside down on a paper towel.
- Store in a clean dry area.
- In hospital each set should be clearly labelled with the mother's name and identifying number.
- The surface of the electronic pump should be cleaned in the same way.
- In the hospital all pumps should be serviced at regular intervals.

Storage of expressed breastmilk

As described in Chapter 2, breastmilk is a 'living fluid', containing antibodies, and anti-infective properties such as IgA, lysosomes, lactoferrin and white blood cells. Therefore, the recommendations for storage of breastmilk are significantly different from those for formula milk (see Table 3.3). All mothers should be advised to wash their hands thoroughly before expressing breastmilk and to wash containers (preferably glass or hard plastic with a lid) with hot soapy water, rinse and allow to air dry before use. Containers should be labelled with the date (and name, particularly if storing breastmilk away from the home). To avoid waste, only the required amounts should be stored in each container, for example 50–100ml. The containers should have enough space left to allow for the breastmilk to expand when frozen.

However, in the neonatal unit additional precautions must be taken. Mothers who are hand expressing should use sterile containers to collect breastmilk (such as an enteral syringe or gallipots) and stored with the infant's name, unit number, date and time the milk was expressed. Sterile bottles should be used when using a breast pump, which should be labelled as above. It is advisable not to overfill the bottles as there could be wastage.

TABLE 3.3 The storage of breastmilk

Storage	Temperature (°C)	Time
Room temperature	19 to 26	4 to 8 hours
Refrigerator	≤4	3 to 8 days
	5 to 10	3 days
Freezer	=18 to 20	6 to 12 months

Sources: BFN (2009a); adapted from La Leche League International (2009).

Reheating and defrosting breastmilk

Breastmilk should not be warmed using direct heat or a microwave. A microwave does not heat the milk evenly and can cause 'hot spots' in the milk. It can also destroy some of the breastmilk's properties. Breastmilk can be warmed in a container of warm water or the container placed under warm running water for a few minutes. Frozen breastmilk can either be left in the fridge to defrost or placed under cool running water. Once thawed, it can be stored in the refrigerator for 12–24 hours (BFN, 2009a; La Leche League International, 2009). Mothers sometimes describe a change in appearance of breastmilk when stored due to the separation of the casein and whey. Once shaken this will rectify itself.

Storage of breastmilk in the neonatal unit

In the neonatal unit breastmilk should be stored in a fridge designated for this purpose only. Temperature recordings should be taken daily and should not exceed 2–4°C. Expressed breastmilk should be used within 24 hours or frozen in a freezer at a temperature of –20°C for a maximum of six months.

Concluding comments

In order to meet the WHO recommendations of exclusive breastfeeding for six months and to continue for two years and beyond, healthcare professionals must develop the knowledge and skills to support, advise and empower breastfeeding mothers. This chapter has covered the basic skills required to do this. Without effective position and attachment the breasts will not be emptied effectively, leading to a build-up of FIL and a decrease in milk supply. Many mothers suggest they discontinue breastfeeding because of insufficient milk supply. Poor position and attachment are the main reasons for this problem and the consequential unsettled infant and, in some cases, extreme weight loss and failure to thrive. In 2010, the BFI recommended that all mothers should have a breastfeeding assessment at day 5 and that this should include assessment of milk transfer.

Hand expression and the safe storage of breastmilk are also basic skills that healthcare professionals must be able to teach mothers, in order to empower them to solve their own problems should they arise. Good communication skills are crucial in transferring this knowledge in a way mothers can understand and remember; therefore both verbal and written information should be provided for all mothers.

Quiz

1   Name the six principles of good positioning.
2   What position might you recommend for a mother to hold her infant to breastfeed following a Caesarean section?
3   Name five signs of effective attachment to the breast.
4   Name three signs of ineffective attachment.
5   When is the fat content of the feed at its highest?
6   When do BFI recommend all breastfeeding mothers should have a feeding assessment and why?
7   How can you assess adequate milk transfer?
8   If separated from the infant how many times a day should the mother express breastmilk?
9   Describe the technique of hand expression.
10 Why would you recommend a mother to 'double pump'?

Resources

*   Department of Health
        www.dh.gov.uk/publications
*   Growth chart information
        www.growthcharts.rcpch.ac.uk
        www.who.int/childgrowth/en
*   Suzanne Colson's Biological Nurturing
        www.biologicalnurturing.com

Chapter 4 **Good practice to promote, initiate and support breastfeeding**

- Learning outcomes
- Breastfeeding policy
- Education and training for healthcare professionals
- Antenatal preparation
- Skin-to-skin contact
- Teaching a mother to maintain lactation
- Avoiding supplements
- Recognising infant feeding cues
- Demand feeding
- Avoiding teats and dummies
- Support groups
- Concluding comments
- Scenarios
- Quiz
- Further reading

Renfrew *et al.* (2000, p. 15) conducted a systematic review of interventions that support or interfere with breastfeeding and identified the following 'key practice areas' that supported breastfeeding:

- a positive informed attitude to breastfeeding;
- effective positioning and attachment;
- pain-free, effective feeding;
- flexible patterns of feeding;
- no routine use of bottles, teats, dummies and nipple shields;
- evidence-based practice in maternity units.

The BFI focuses on the key practice areas and implementation of the Baby Friendly best practice standards has been identified as one way to increase breastfeeding rates (Tappin *et al.*, 2001; Britten and Broadfoot, 2002; Broadfoot *et al.*, 2005a; Merten *et al.*, 2005; DiGirolamo *et al.*, 2008). Merten *et al.* (2005) suggest that the increases in breastfeeding rates in Switzerland since 1994 are in part a result of the increasing numbers of healthcare facilities accredited as 'Baby Friendly'. Infants born in accredited facilities had a longer duration of breastfeeding than those born in facilities without accreditation. They attributed this to compliance with the *Ten Steps*. This chapter will focus on evidence-based good practice to promote and support breastfeeding based on the *Ten Steps to Successful Breastfeeding* and the *Seven Point Plan*, as well as practices that may interfere with successful breastfeeding.

Learning outcomes

By the end of this chapter you will be able to:

* identify evidence-based practice that will promote, initiate and support breastfeeding;
* avoid practices that interfere with successful breastfeeding;
* provide individualised education and support to help mothers initiate and maintain lactation.

Mapping the UNICEF UK BFI educational outcomes

5 Understand the potential impact of delivery room practices on the well-being of mother and baby and on the establishment of breastfeeding in particular.

6 Understand why it is important for mothers to keep their babies near them.

7 Understand the principle of demand feeding and be able to explain its importance in relation to the establishment and maintenance of lactation.

8 Be equipped to provide parents with accurate, evidence-based information about activities that may have an impact on breastfeeding.

9 Understand the importance of exclusive breastfeeding for the first six months of life and possess the knowledge and skills to enable mothers to achieve this.

Breastfeeding policy

> **STEP 1/POINT 1**: Have a written breastfeeding policy that is routinely communicated to all healthcare staff.

Step 1/Point 1 states that healthcare facilities should have a written breast-feeding policy that is routinely communicated to all healthcare staff (UNICEF, 2001). During the BFI accreditation process, healthcare facilities have to demonstrate that all staff involved in providing care for breastfeeding mothers comply with the policy. The policy should identify the aims, principles and standards to be achieved, ensuring that staff adhere to the WHO Code (1981). The policy should be supported by guidelines on how to implement it, including the evidence-based management of common complications. Having a policy ensures commitment from managers and administrators to implement practices that promote, support and protect breastfeeding. It also encourages a consistent approach between doctors, midwives, health visitors and other staff leading to a reduction in conflicting advice.

The WHO (1998a) recommended that policies are developed by the multiagency team and should:

- be specific to breastfeeding rather than general obstetric policies;
- include aims and objectives;
- specify practices that promote breastfeeding such as 'rooming-in' and avoiding supplementary feeds without medical indication;
- adhere to the *Ten Steps*, WHO Code and WHA recommendations;
- include local and national breastfeeding rates;
- include referral pathways.

All staff supporting breastfeeding mothers should be orientated to the policy and Step 2/Point 2 states that, within six months of employment, healthcare staff should receive training and education to implement the policy. The policy should also be audited at regular intervals to ensure it is having the desired effect, and that all staff are adhering to it.

Education and training for healthcare professionals

> **STEP 2/POINT 2**: Train all healthcare staff in skills necessary to implement the policy.

Healthcare professionals' lack of knowledge and skills to support mothers to breastfeed their infants have been identified as a major contributing factor in low rates of initiation and duration of breastfeeding, leading to inconsistent and inaccurate advice (Sikorski *et al.*, 2002; Hall-Moran *et al.*, 2004; Renfrew *et al.*, 2005). Evidence suggests this may be due to a lack of formal education opportunities and 'chaotic' learning environments (Renfrew *et al.*, 2005; Smale *et al.*, 2006; Jackson, 2007; McFadden *et al.*, 2007). It therefore cannot be assumed that all professionals have the knowledge and skills to provide adequate support and advice for mothers.

There appears to be a consensus that, in order to ensure health professionals provide competent and confident support for mothers who breastfeed their infants, provision of effective education and training is essential in under-graduate programmes as well as continuous professional development (UNICEF, 2001; Cantrill *et al.*, 2003; DH, 2004b; Renfrew *et al.*, 2005; Ingram, 2006; NICE, 2006a; Jackson, 2007; McFadden *et al.*, 2007). Renfrew *et al.* (2005) conducted a multidisciplinary breastfeeding knowledge and skills assessment, which claimed that, as well as a deficit in formal breastfeeding education, there was also a lack of infrastructure to support breastfeeding education within the clinical setting. Apart from the UNICEF BFI (2001) they found that there were few formal learning opportunities, including a lack of provision of breastfeeding education via HE institutions. Participants in this study expressed concern that this was having a direct effect on care provision as professionals were giving mothers inconsistent advice based on a lack of knowledge.

There have been several studies that have demonstrated that structured evidence-based training programmes for healthcare professionals increase confidence, knowledge and skill. For example, Ingram (2006), who introduced a CD-ROM breastfeeding learning package to primary care teams, use a questionnaire to assess attitudes, knowledge and management of breastfeeding. She found an improvement in all areas for each professional group and reported improvements in care. These findings are supported by Kronborg *et al.* (2007), who suggested that introducing an interactive programme for health visitors improved their knowledge and self-efficacy.

Tappin *et al.* (2006) conducted a cross-sectional study in Glasgow in 2000 to explore health visitors' intervention, activities and attitudes towards breast-feeding. A significant finding of this study was that mothers who were breast-feeding at the first health visitor's visit were more likely to still be breastfeeding at the second routine visit if the health visitor had been trained in support-ing breastfeeding mothers within the last two years. They suggested that an evidence-based programme similar to the BFI breastfeeding management course would be appropriate, but recognised the need for further research in this area.

The BFI (UNICEF, 2002, 2008b) recommend a minimum of 18 hours of breastfeeding education throughout midwifery and health visitors' programmes to rectify this problem before students become registered practitioners. This is supported by Dodgson and Tarrant (2007), who conducted a study to deter-mine the effectiveness of an infant feeding educational intervention on student nurses in the USA. The intervention group received ten hours of didactic teaching and an eight-week clinical placement. They found that the intervention group scored higher on the knowledge survey than the control group and more readily associated breastfeeding with a positive maternal and child outcome. Despite this increase in knowledge, the mean score was only 54.3 per cent, comparable to a similar study conducted by Spear (2004), demonstrating that more work needs to be done. Dodgson and Tarrant (2007) suggest revisiting and integrating infant feeding education in other courses where appropriate. The majority of students in this study reported that they would be more likely to promote breastfeeding using evidence-based knowledge and less likely to practise in ways that could be detrimental to successful breastfeeding.

Employers have questioned why midwives and health visitors are exiting their educational programmes without the essential knowledge or skills for practice (UNICEF, 2002, 2009). In response to this criticism, the UNICEF UK BFI developed the *Best Practice Standards for Higher Education Institutions*, along with an accreditation procedure (UNICEF, 2002) (see Appendix 1).

Antenatal preparation

> **STEP 3/POINT 3**: Inform all pregnant women about the benefits and manage-ment of breastfeeding.

Attending for antenatal care is related to better breastfeeding outcomes (Bolling *et al.*, 2007; SACN, 2008). The *Infant Feeding Survey 2005* (Bolling *et al.*, 2007) highlights that choice of infant method is influenced by culture, education and socio-economic background, including the attitudes of partners, other relatives, friends and healthcare professionals. For some, becoming pregnant may be the first time they have considered the issue of infant feeding. It may also be the first time they have received any evidence-based information on infant feeding practices. One of the aims of antenatal education is to inform pregnant women about the benefits of breastfeeding to help them be successful and avoid problems.

Advantages of antenatal education are that it:

- provides mothers with knowledge to make informed choices;
- increases confidence;
- increases breastfeeding rates;
- dispels myths.

The BFI recommends that all mothers are offered written information and one-to-one information about the benefits and management of breastfeeding before 34 weeks' gestation, as well as the opportunity to attend a breastfeeding workshop (even if a mother has been admitted to hospital within this time) (UNICEF, 2010e). As well as teaching the pregnant woman about the anatomy and physiology of breastfeeding, more specific issues should be discussed such as skin-to-skin contact; rooming-in or 'keeping baby close'; avoiding supplements; and demand feeding (feeding when the baby shows signs of wanting to feed) (UNICEF, 2010e). It is also important to address myths and inhibitions surrounding breastfeeding. Baby Friendly hospitals have a checklist to ensure that all women are given this information so that they can make an informed choice about infant feeding.

Women should also be given advice about how to successfully initiate and continue breastfeeding at this time. Some clinicians advise antenatal expression of colostrum to increase the duration of breastfeeding and reduce the incidence of engorgement and sore nipples. However, in a systematic review Renfrew *et al.* (2000) found a dearth of available evidence to support this practice and recommend it should be a matter of personal choice. Some clinicians recommend antenatal expression of breastmilk to mothers who are at risk of preterm birth or whose infants are high risk and may have difficulty breastfeeding initially (see Chapters 6 and 7). The intention is that the infant can receive expressed colostrum if supplementation is required instead of formula milk. This process can commence at around 36 weeks of pregnancy, but stopped if any uterine contractions or tightening are felt. The procedure is the same as for the expression of milk (see Chapter 3). However, colostrum will only be expressed in small amounts and should be collected in small sterile syringes or other suitable receptacles so that none of it is wasted. If colostrum is expressed more than once a day a new receptacle should be used each time. The colostrum should be frozen at −18°C and labelled appropriately. If the mother is bringing it into hospital it will require a name, date and identifying number.

Some women are also encouraged to prepare their nipples to 'toughen' them in preparation for breastfeeding. Once again, Renfrew *et al.* (2000) found no evidence to support this practice; however, they did suggest that a possible benefit could be to prepare mothers to feel confident when handling their breasts.

Skin-to-skin contact

> **STEP 4**: Help mothers initiate breastfeeding soon after birth.

Despite differences of the timing of the first breastfeed in different cultures, it is strongly recommended that it should take place as soon as possible following birth. Unhurried skin-to-skin contact is one way of encouraging this and it should not be interrupted to provide routine care such as weighing the infant or bathing. Where mother and infant are separated for clinical reasons, skin-to-skin contact should commence as soon as mother and infant are able to do so. During unrestricted skin-to-skin, in the first hour following birth, oxytocin levels are high (Nissen *et al.*, 1996), which, as well as encouraging the let-down reflex, facilitates instinctive breastfeeding behaviour in both the mother and the infant or, as described by Nils Bergman (2008), the neuro-behavioural programme. Moore *et al.* (2009) conducted a systematic review of 30 studies, including 1,925 mother–infant dyads. They found that infants who had skin-to-skin contact interacted more with their mothers, maintained their temperature and cried less. They were also more likely to breastfeed and for a longer duration (see Figure 4.1).

If infants are separated from their mothers they display signs of '*hyper-arousal response*', where the heart rate, respiratory rate and blood pressure increase (Bergman, 2008), even if this is in a cot in the same room. They cry much more than usual, in short pulses, which is possibly a distress call for the mother as exhibited in other mammals (WHO, 1998a) and which may impair lung and cardiac function.

The *Infant Feeding Survey 2005* (Bolling *et al.*, 2007) reported that only 72 per cent of mothers in the UK had skin-to-skin contact with their infants within an hour of birth and that initiation of breastfeeding was higher for those exposed to skin-to-skin; 87 per cent of those mothers breastfed within one hour of birth. The survey also identified a link between delayed initiation of breastfeeding and early cessation.

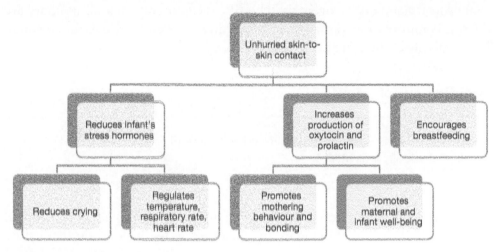

FIGURE 4.1 The benefits of skin-to-skin contact

The BFI also recommends that all mothers should be offered help with the first breastfeed within six hours of birth (UNICEF, 2010e); however, Bolling *et al.* (2007) reported that only seven in ten mothers had been shown how to put their infant to the breast in the first few days.

Narcotics administered during labour may interfere with the first feed as they affect the breastfeeding behaviour of the infant; side effects include shorter periods of wakefulness; poor sucking; being less alert to social stimuli and ultimately a delay in effective feeding (Walker, 2010). Consideration must be given to the impact on breastfeeding when recommending routine use of analgesia in labour and following birth. Infants of these mothers should be kept in skin-to-skin contact for as long as possible.

Teaching a mother to maintain lactation

STEP 5/POINT 4: Show mothers how to breastfeed and how to maintain lactation, even if they should be separated from their infants.

Many mothers, particularly if they have not breastfed before, need to be shown how to breastfeed and maintain their lactation if separated from their infant. This may include psychological support as well as practical information about technique, such as position and attachment, hand expression and recognising effective milk transfer (see Chapter 3). If the mother and infant are to be separated, it is essential that the mother is taught about hand expression to establish or maintain lactogenesis. The BFI recommends that all mothers are given this information verbally and in writing before they leave the hospital. This is discussed further in Chapter 3.

Avoiding supplements

> **STEP 6/POINT 5**: Give newborn infants no food or drink other than breastmilk, unless medically indicated.

Breastmilk is the natural food for human infants and provides all the nutritional and immunological requirements to meet the individual needs of healthy term infants until the age of six months, and in addition to solid food for two years and beyond (WHO, 2002). Despite the increase in breastfeeding rates, exclusive breastfeeding until six months continues to be a problem. Exclusive breastfeeding is defined as the infant's consumption of human milk with no supplementation of any type (including no water, juice, non-human milk or foods) except for minerals, vitamins and medications (Remmington and Remmington, 2009).

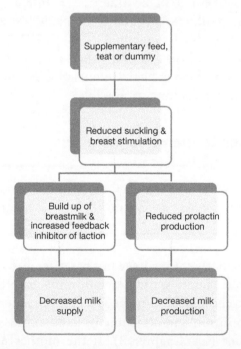

FIGURE 4.2 The effects of supplementary feeds, teats or dummies

The term 'supplementation' can be confusing and often means giving another feed in addition to or in place of a breastfeed, such as formula or even water. The reasons for giving supplementary feeds include medically indicated reasons, lack of evidence-based practice or parental choice and are discussed further in Chapter 8. Unless medically indicated, supplementing breastfeeds should be avoided (Renfrew *et al.*, 2005), because it can increase the risk of allergies and gastrointestinal and respiratory infections, and can encourage premature cessation of breastfeeding (WHO, 1998a). Giving supplements can have an adverse effect on milk supply because it reduces the number of times the breasts are stimulated through suckling to produce prolactin. The ineffective removal of milk will also lead to a build-up of the FIL and ultimately decrease milk production (see Figure 4.2).

The WHO Code (1981) states that mothers should not be given free samples of breastmilk substitutes to take home from hospital because it increases the likelihood that they will bottle feed.

Recognising infant feeding cues

> **STEP 7**: Practise rooming-in: allow mothers and infants to remain together 24 hours a day.

It is important that mothers spend the first few weeks bonding with their infant, learning the infant's feeding cues and behaviour. Crying is considered a late sign of hunger and it is important to teach the mother earlier signs that her infant needs to breastfeed (Both and Frischknect, 2008). Feeding cues may include the following:

- sucking movements;
- sucking noises;
- lip licking;
- head movement from side to side;
- rapid eye movements;
- restlessness.

Rooming-in

In the past most hospitals practised 'nursery care' for infants. The intention was often altruistic but it had negative consequences for breastfeeding. Nursery care was justified by midwives, who said they were taking the infant away to let the mother rest; however, evidence suggests that mothers actually sleep better when with their infant due to the oxytocin release (Ball, 2003). The separated infant was also at risk of receiving supplementary feeds and dummies and this practice also increased the risk of infection and deprived the mother–infant dyad the opportunity to interact and develop innate feeding behaviour, maternal feelings and confidence (WHO, 1998a). In contrast, 'rooming-in', or keeping the mother and infant together, enables the mother to get to know her infant, learn the feeding cues and gain confidence in handling the infant. It facilitates unrestricted feeds, which in turn stimulates production of prolactin and empties the breasts regularly. If the mother learns her infant's feeding cues, she can react quickly and breastfeed the infant before it becomes too distressed and more difficult to attach to the breast.

Bed-sharing

Current Department of Health advice recommends that the safest place for infants to sleep is in their own cot in the same room as the parents. However, bed-sharing promotes breastfeeding and breastfeeding reduces the risk of sudden infant death syndrome (SIDS) (Vennemann *et al.*, 2009). Bed-sharing is a contentious issue and often places the promotion of breastfeeding and the prevention of SIDS in conflict. An example of this was the inaccurate media reports on the case-control study conducted in 2009 by Blair *et al*. The media claimed bed-sharing for breastfeeding was contraindicated. The aim of the study had been to ascertain the major risk factors associated with SIDS in 0–2 year olds. It was conducted over a four-year period in the southwest of England and concluded that many of the SIDS infants had co-slept in a hazardous environment and that the major influences were parental use of alcohol or drugs prior to co-sleeping, or sleeping on the sofa. They suggested that these factors could be addressed by educating parents not to fall asleep with the infant on the sofa and not to co-sleep if they had taken drugs or alcohol.

Helen Ball is a well-known anthropologist who has done a large amount of research into bed-sharing and co-sleeping. She states (Ball, 2009) that anthropologists consider mother–infant sleep as normal for humans and recent research confirms that bed-sharing is common practice. Ball (2002, 2003) conducted a study with 253 families in the northwest of England and reported that 47 per cent slept in the same bed as their one-month-old infant, but this figure dropped to 29 per cent when the infant was three months old. These findings were supported by the *Infant Feeding Survey 2005* (Bolling *et al.*, 2007). Ball (2003) suggests that mothers who share a bed with their infant in the first month are twice as likely to be breastfeeding at four months of age. In 2006, Ball *et al*. conducted a randomised trial of infant sleep location on the postnatal ward. They videoed mother–infant dyads in different locations:

(1) the infant in a normal cot by the bed; (2) the infant in a side cot attached to the bed; and (3) with the infant in the bed with cot sides. They observed that those infants in the side cot or in bed attempted to and successfully breastfed more frequently than those in the standard cot by the bed. The ability to root and suckle was hampered for those infants in standard cots and the mothers were unable to see the feeding cues readily, or their responses were hindered by not being able to access the cot easily and sometimes requiring assistance.

Ball *et al.* (2006) also observed differences in sleep positions between breastfeeding mothers and formula-feeding mothers. Breastfeeding mothers adopted a protective position more often than formula-feeding mothers. They slept facing the infant, on their side with their legs curled under the infant's feet, protecting the infant from some of the above risks. The infant's position was level to the breast within the space created by the mother. Formula-feeding mothers spent more time asleep turned away from their infants.

As discussed in Chapter 2, it is important that mothers respond early to feeding cues, particularly in the first few days, to ensure adequate production of prolactin to prime the lactocytes, in order to initiate and maintain lactation (lactogenesis II). Night-time feeds are particularly important as greater amounts of prolactin are released.

Key fact

Prolactin levels peak at night (circadian rhythm) and therefore night feeds must be encouraged to promote milk production.

The benefits of sharing a bed are well documented in terms of physical and psychological development and include:

- regulation of breathing, heart rate and thermoregulation;
- improvement of breastfeeding initiation and duration by increasing the frequency of breastfeeds during the night when prolactin levels peak;
- enabling the mother to respond quickly to infant feeding cues;
- reduction in the incidence of SIDS;
- reduction in the incidence of neglect;
- an increased feeling of closeness and bonding.

However, safety is paramount and parents must be given information about risk factors associated with bed-sharing that increase the risk of SIDS and how to reduce the risk of accidents or overheating. In 2008, UNICEF BFI developed a leaflet, 'Sharing a bed with your baby', in collaboration with the Foundation for the Study of Infant Deaths (www.babyfriendly.org.uk/pdfs/sharingbed leaflet.pdf). It includes the following advice for parents:

- **Never** lie with or co-sleep on the sofa or in an armchair.
- **Do Not sleep with the baby if:**
  - you or your partner smoke;
  - you or your partner have taken alcohol or drugs (legal or illegal), are ill or unusually tired, or if the infant is unwell and has a high temperature;
  - the infant was premature or small for gestational age.

If parents choose to bed-share they must be given information to enable them to reduce the risk of accidents or overheating:

- The mattress should be firm (no waterbeds).
- Ensure the infant cannot become trapped between the bed and the wall or fall out of bed.
- Do not overdress the infant.
- Do not leave the infant alone in bed.
- The room must not be too hot; 16–18°C is ideal.
- Bedding must not cover the infant's head.
- Ensure the partner knows when the infant is taken into bed.
- If there is another child in the bed, ensure an adult is between them.
- Pets should not share the bed.

Demand feeding

> **STEP 8**: Encourage breastfeeding on demand.

Restricting infant feeds was introduced in the early twentieth century in an attempt to make breastfeeding more scientific. It was thought that the infant's stomach needed three to four hours to empty and that prolonged feeding could cause problems such as diarrhoea and vomiting. It is now widely accepted that restricting breastfeeds can lead to an insufficient milk supply, failure to thrive (due to not getting the high fat content milk at the end of a feed) and early cessation of breastfeeding.

Mothers should be encouraged to recognise feeding cues and, unless clinically indicated, breastfeed their infants on demand. This is referred to as demand feeding, unrestricted or baby-led feeding. Demand feeding means that no restrictions should be made on the frequency and duration of feeds. If there is concern in the early days after birth about the length of time between feeds, the mother may need to wake the infant up and encourage it to feed to establish or maintain lactation to avoid a build-up of the FIL, which will cause inhibition of milk production. It is also important for the mother to avoid her breasts becoming too full and uncomfortable, leading to engorgement, blocked ducts or mastitis.

Parents are often concerned about time limits and should be advised that every infant's requirements will be different. However, on average, infants should breastfeed about eight times in a 24-hour period. They may find at some times in the day that the infant will cluster feed and then go for longer periods at another time. There may be medical requirements where the infant's condition does not allow demand feeding and it needs to feed frequently and regularly. However, as soon as possible, demand feeding should be encouraged.

While in hospital, it is important that hospital routines and procedures do not interfere with demand feeding (such as meal times, examination, ward rounds). Also, in the home visitors should not disrupt this process. Some mothers find visitors keen to come and help with the infant; however, it would be more beneficial if they helped with domestic chores and allowed the mother and infant to be together.

The benefits of demand feeding include:

* maintaining an adequate milk supply;
* less infant weight loss in the immediate postpartum period;
* increased duration of breastfeeding;
* prevention of engorgement, blocked ducts and mastitis;
* reduction in hyperbilirubinaemia (elevation of bilirubin levels causing jaundice).

Avoiding teats and dummies

STEP 9: Give no artificial teats or dummies to breastfeeding infants.

Nipple confusion can be defined as the interference of artificial nipples such as teats and pacifiers/dummies with the successful initiation of breastfeeding.

The use of dummies/pacifiers is common practice in the UK and the recommendation by BFI to avoid their use has been a contentious issue among mothers and healthcare professionals (Renfrew *et al.*, 2000). This argument was exacerbated by the inclusion of dummies as a preventative measure against cot death in 2007, by the Foundation for the Study of Infant Deaths (FSID, 2009). FSID suggested that providing a dummy to settle the infant to sleep, even for naps, could prevent cot death. However, it did add that, if breastfeeding, the dummy should not be introduced until the infant is one month old and breastfeeding is well established.

Hargreaves and Harris (2009) argue that the evidence to support the avoidance of teats or dummies in healthy term infants is limited and much of the research to support this idea is based on premature infants or infants with other compounding factors. They suggest midwives should adopt a more flexible and woman-centred approach when advising mothers. The BFI recognised this, and the need for flexibility within the neonatal unit, and has since removed this standard from the formal assessment on neonatal units during hospital assessments (UNICEF, 2010e). Renfrew *et al.* (2005) also highlighted the lack of good research and recommended further research in this area. They suggested that the problem of nipple confusion could be better termed 'acquired teat preference', suggesting that individual infants prefer one nipple/teat above another.

The main problem with introducing teats or dummies appears to exist within the first few weeks following birth, as breastfeeding is becoming established, and is associated with the following problems:

- altered suck-swallow-breathe cycle, and lower oxygen saturation in preterm infants;
- reduced number of breastfeeds per day;
- decrease in milk production due to lack of breast stimulation (see Figure 4.2, page 72);
- early cessation of breastfeeding;
- increase in tooth decay;
- increase in ear infections;
- potential introduction of candida albicans (thrush).

The BFI recommends that, where supplementary feeds are necessary, an alternative method of feeding is used, such as cup feeding, to avoid artificial teats; this is discussed further in Chapter 8.

Support groups

> **STEP 10/POINTS 6,7**: Identify sources of national and local support for breast-feeding and ensure that mothers know how to access these prior to discharge from hospital.

It is important that breastfeeding mothers do not feel isolated when they leave the hospital, and in recent years there have been a number of initiatives developed to provide support in the community; however, many still require evaluation. It is therefore important to provide mothers with information about the types of support they can access and how to do this. This can be done in the form of a list of contact telephone numbers or websites for midwives, health visitors, support groups (lay and professionals), peer supporters and coun-sellors. In 2010, the BFI introduced the requirement for hospitals to provide both written and verbal information about national and local support for both stages 1 and 3 of the hospital accreditation process. Sources of community support are further explored in Chapter 10.

Concluding comments

The BFI standards are a good point of reference to identify practices that will either support or interfere with successful breastfeeding and have been shown to improve breastfeeding rates (Broadfoot *et al.*, 2005b; Merten *et al.*, 2005). However, it has to be acknowledged that a great deal more robust research is required to support many areas of practice. Mothers need to be empowered with the correct 'toolkit' from the birth of their infant to give them confidence to breastfeed for as long as they choose to, which includes practical skills as well as evidence-based information.

Practice should be developed to meet the needs of the mother and infant rather than organisational processes. Steps 1 and 2 are probably most funda-mental in this respect. It is crucial that there is a health board/authority strategy and policy that has commitment from the executive team and managers and that all relevant healthcare professionals receive adequate training, preferably in the pre-registration programme, but also as part of their continuous professional development. By doing this, healthcare professionals will be able to provide consistent and accurate information for mothers and infants in their care. This chapter has explored how this can be achieved and potential problems avoided. The following chapter will explore more specific problems individual mothers may encounter and how they can be resolved.

Scenarios

1   Jane is 42 and gave birth to her baby 11 days ago. Her baby has lost 10 per cent of its birthweight. Her life is hectic and her other children are four years old and 18 months. The baby is described as a 'crying, fretful baby' and you have implemented good practice for improving weight gain, effective positioning and attachment, and hand expressing.

Jane asks you about skin-to-skin contact and guidance on safe bed-sharing:

• **How would you advise Jane?**

2   Joanne is an 18-year-old prim who has had a rotational forceps delivery of a 4.87kg male infant. Labour was documented as lasting 26 hours with an active pushing stage of nearly two hours. Joanne had a 1.8 litre blood loss and has been in High Dependency for the last eight hours following the birth. The baby is very bruised and unsettled and has been feeding frequently. Positioning and attachment have been noted as 'good' and Joanne is requesting that the baby be taken away as she is exhausted.

You are looking after Joanne:

• **What would you say to Joanne?**
• **What can you do to help her?**
• **What can you do for the baby?**

Quiz

1   Give three reasons why a normal healthy term baby may not feed regularly within the first 24–48 hours.
2   Name four benefits of skin-to-skin contact.
3   List the ways parents can reduce the risk of overheating and accidents if they choose to bed-share.
4   Why is 'rooming-in' recommended?
5   What are the advantages of having a breastfeeding policy for mothers?
6   How can you inform mothers about the breastfeeding policy in your area of practice?
7   What advice would you give a mother who suggests she is going to give her baby a dummy?
8   How would you explain what is meant by demand feeding?
9   Why should supplementary feeds not be given to breastfeeding infants?
10 Describe the infant feeding cues you should teach mothers to look out for.

Further reading

- UNICEF (2010) *Hospital Initiative Review 2010*, London: UNICEF.
- Breastfeeding Care Pathways
  www.babyfriendly.org.uk/pdfs/dh_hp_breastfeeding_care_
  pathway.pdf
  www.babyfriendly.org.uk/pdfs/dh_mothers_breastfeeding_
  journey.pdf

Chapter 5 **Management of common problems**

- Learning outcomes
- Lactation history
- Insufficient milk supply
- Nipple pain or trauma
- Inverted nipples
- Breast engorgement
- Blocked ducts
- Mastitis
- Abscesses
- Thrush or candida albicans
- Breast refusal
- Concluding comments
- Scenarios
- Resources

Many mothers will experience common complications of breastfeeding and will require skilled support and advice to ensure that lactation continues. Following on from the basic skills required to support breastfeeding mothers in Chapter 3, and how to promote good practice to support and protect breastfeeding in Chapter 4, this chapter addresses the knowledge and skills required to support mothers with some of the common problems they may experience. It builds on the skills of how to observe effective milk transfer discussed in Chapter 3, beginning with the fundamental skill of taking a detailed lactation history to identify the root of the problem so that it may be corrected. However, it must be remembered that each mother is an individual and the management must be skilfully tailored to meet her needs and those of the infant.

Learning outcomes

By the end of this chapter you will be able to:

* take an accurate lactation history;
* identify the common complications of breastfeeding;
* diagnose the common complications of breastfeeding;
* teach a mother how to avoid the common complications of breastfeeding;
* describe safe and effective techniques and treatments for the common complications of breastfeeding.

Mapping the UNICEF UK BFI educational outcomes

15 Know about the common complications of breastfeeding, how these arise and how women may be helped to overcome them.

Lactation history

It is acknowledged that problems with breastfeeding can be the result of psychosocial and physical issues, as well as hospital practices, poor advice and a lack of support from healthcare professionals. Therefore, taking a lactation or breastfeeding history alongside an observation of a complete breastfeed is essential to get to the root of the problem and to be able to make an accurate diagnosis. The BFI (UNICEF, 2008a) has developed a comprehensive breast-feeding history form (see Appendix 4), which contains a systematic series of questions to explore the possible situations that may interfere with successful breastfeeding, so that an appropriate and individualised plan of care can be developed. It includes questions on the following areas:

1 **Current feeding situation**: Exploring the current feeding pattern, use of supplements or dummies/pacifiers, milk expression and any separation of mother and infant.
2 **Infant's current health and behaviour**: Exploring the infant's feeding behaviour and general health (including weight and urine and stool output).
3 **The early postnatal period**: Exploring the infant's condition at birth, and early care and hospital practices, such as the opportunity for skin-to-skin contact, rooming-in, or any supplements previously given.
4 **Pregnancy and birth**: Exploring pregnancy issues and preparation for breastfeeding, and relevant labour and birth issues, including analgesia, blood loss, intact placenta and membranes.

5 **Mother's health**: Exploring general health, disabilities, medical conditions, medication, smoking, alcohol usage and family planning.

6 **Previous experience of breastfeeding.**

7 **Family and social situation**: Exploring support from the partner, family and friends, help with domestic chores and returning to work.

Good communication skills are key to obtaining an accurate history as discussed in Chapter 11.

Key facts

For all breastfeeding problems:

1 Take a lactation history.

2 Observe a complete breastfeed for effective milk transfer:

✔ correct position and attachment;

✔ sucking pattern.

3 Observe for breast or nipple anomalies.

4 Assess the infant's mouth for tongue-tie or any other anomaly.

5 Encourage skin-to-skin contact.

6 Use positive language to promote confidence.

7 Produce a care plan to avoid conflicting advice.

Insufficient milk supply

A common concern for breastfeeding mothers is whether their infants are getting enough milk. This is often due to a lack of confidence as a result of influences inherent in a bottle-feeding culture, where the amounts of formula milk are measured and regulated. Insufficient milk supply is often cited by mothers as a reason for early weaning or giving up breastfeeding (Gatti, 2008). In a large study of 1,323 mothers who completed questionnaires at regular intervals between two and twelve months following birth, Li *et al.* (2008) found that one of the most common reasons for stopping breastfeeding was the mother's perception that she did not have enough milk to satisfy the infant. This view was particularly prevalent in low-income groups. The role of the healthcare professional is therefore crucial in recognising the difference between perceived insufficient milk supply or physiologically delayed or failed lactogenesis, to ensure mothers have the tools to give them confidence to rectify the problem and continue breastfeeding.

Physical, psychological and social factors can affect lactogenesis. Failed lactation can be classified as primary or secondary:

- **Primary** inability to produce breastmilk.
- **Secondary** due to poor techniques or management of breastfeeding problems.

Some common causes of failed lactation are hormonal imbalance due to conditions such as diabetes, hypothyroidism and obesity (Hurst, 2007). Birthing complications such as preterm birth, Caesarean section and retained placenta may also be contributing factors. Other issues that may cause problems are breast trauma, surgery, anxiety or stress, postpartum haemorrhage leading to Sheehan's syndrome, and polycystic ovaries. However, failed lactogenesis is most commonly associated with a lack of skin-to-skin contact, infrequent feeding and ineffective removal of milk from the breast for a variety of reasons, such as tongue-tie, maternal–infant separation, poor attachment, supplementary feeds, and use of teats and pacifiers. The combined contraceptive pill and other medications can also inhibit milk production. This list is by no means exhaustive and these and other issues are further discussed throughout this book.

Hurst (2007) suggested that the presence of two or more of the following risk factors for delay or failure of lactation should indicate close surveillance of the initiation of breastfeeding for signs of adequate milk supply and transfer, such as frequent wet nappies and changing stool (see Chapter 3). Signs of inadequate milk transfer are:

- fewer than three wet nappies per day by the third day;
- fewer than six wet nappies per day by the fifth day;
- no evidence of 'changing' stools by the third or fourth day;
- further weight loss after the third day or a weight loss of greater than 7 per cent of the birthweight;
- poor weight gain;
- infant not satiated;
- soft breasts;
- no signs of milk transfer during feed (swallowing signs, visible milk);
- persistent jaundice.

Recognising the problem at an early stage is crucial and the first steps in supporting mothers with any problems associated with breastfeeding are:

- to observe a complete breastfeed (see Chapter 3);
- to take a lactation history:

  - frequency of feeds and feeding pattern;
  - use of supplementary feeds, teats or dummies;
  - birth history;
  - number of wet nappies and consistency/colour of stools.

Once the reason for the inadequate milk supply has been identified, a plan of action can be developed, implemented and evaluated. The focus of this plan should be to ensure adequate nutrition for the infant and to increase breast stimulation and effective emptying of breastmilk. This can be achieved by:

1 Skin-to skin contact.
2 Increasing the number of times the mother breastfeeds per day, ensuring at least one feed during the night. 'Switch' feeding may keep the infant awake (changing from one breast to the other several times during a feed on a short-term basis).
3 If supplementation is required because of failure to thrive, ideally breastmilk should be given, rather than formula milk, following a breastfeed. This should be delivered using devices other than a bottle or teat to avoid nipple–teat confusion (see Chapter 8).
4 Teaching the mother to correct any positioning and attachment problems (see Chapter 3).
5 Rectifying any problems such as tongue-tie (see Chapter 7).
6 Additional breast stimulation and complete breast emptying using a mechanical breast pump (see Chapter 3).
7 If required, use of galactagogues such as domperidone and metoclopramide to increase prolactin levels (see Chapter 7).

Nipple pain or trauma

Painful nipples are one of the most common reasons for mothers stopping breastfeeding (Lewallen *et al.*, 2006). Nipples may feel sensitive and tender in the early days of breastfeeding but should not be painful. Painful nipples may be associated with sore or cracked nipples, which may have a fissure, blisters and bleeding. If the mother complains of pain in the first few days it is likely be a problem with positioning and attachment (Albright, 2003). However, pain can also be a symptom of thrush and other problems, which should be ruled out (these conditions will be discussed later in this chapter). An open wound in the nipple is also a portal of entry for infection. Other reasons for nipple pain could be Raynaud's disease, eczema, dermatitis or impetigo (Albright, 2003).

Raynaud's disease is caused by the short-term but exaggerated vaso-constriction of blood vessels, usually in the extremities such as fingers and toes, leading to hypoxia of the tissue. Raynaud's disease can also be found in the nipple and is a treatable condition, but it is often mistaken for thrush because of the severe pain (Anderson *et al.*, 2004). It is associated with cold temperatures and causes blanching of the nipple and sometimes cyanosis or erythema (redness of the skin). Anderson *et al.* (2004) recommend that diagnosis is made when biphasic (cyanosis and erythema) or triphasic (pallor, cyanosis, erythema) colour changes of the nipple are noted. Mothers with this condition may also have experienced these symptoms during pregnancy and when not breastfeeding. Treatment includes avoiding cold temperatures and substances that cause vasoconstriction, such as nicotine and caffeine. However, because the pain is so severe mothers may need pharmacological intervention, such as nifedipine, which causes vasodilation (Anderson *et al.*, 2004).

Nipple pain can be very distressing for mothers and the resulting anxiety may inhibit the let-down reflex (Lawrence and Lawrence, 2005). It may also lead to reduced frequency and length of breastfeeds or exclusivity of one side, resulting in ineffective removal of breastmilk or even discontinuation of breastfeeding. The aim of treatment is to alleviate the pain while maintaining lactation. Treatment can be difficult because of repeated trauma and potential infection (Lee-Dennis *et al.*, 2009). Therefore, nipples should be assessed and treatment determined on an individual basis. Signs of trauma may include erythema, oedema, blisters, fissures, scabs or bruising under the skin.

A number of interventions have been recommended over the years to treat painful nipples and promote healing to maintain lactation and exclusive breastfeeding, such as ointments, sprays and nipple shields. Nipple shields have caused great controversy for many years and many midwives are wary of suggesting them. In the past, nipple shields were promoted for mothers with sore or cracked nipples, attachment difficulties and 'flat' nipples, without trying to find out the cause of the problem first or teaching the mother about correct positioning and attachment techniques. Nipple shields are thought to reduce milk supply by 22 per cent (Woolridge *et al.*, 1980) and may lead to discontinuation from breastfeeding. In contrast, in a multi-site, international study of 54 maternal–infant dyads using ultra-thin nipple shields, Chertok (2009) found that 89.8 per cent of mothers were satisfied in using them and 67.3 per cent of these mothers suggested that it prevented them giving up breastfeeding. Also, there was no significant difference in weight gain for the infants who fed with or without the nipple shield. This study suggests the judicious use of nipple shields as a temporary measure may be helpful.

Renfrew *et al.* (2005) found a lack of good quality research on treatments for nipple pain and trauma. However, they did suggest the first-line treatment must be to address the most common cause of painful nipples, which is incorrect position and attachment. Caldwell *et al.* (2004) conducted a randomised experimental trial with 94 breastfeeding mothers with sore nipples. They randomly split these mothers into three groups: (1) those who used lanolin and breast shells; (2) those who used glycerine gel dressings; and (3) those who received assessment and education on position and attachment. They found all interventions to be effective, resulting in healed nipples and decreased pain. However, all groups also included assessment and education. Therefore, the authors recommend that care for mothers with sore nipples should include assessment of position and attachment.

Lee-Dennis *et al.* (2009) are currently undertaking a systematic review to assess the effects of all the interventions in the resolution of nipple pain, trauma, infection, maternal satisfaction and breastfeeding exclusivity and duration.

Practice recommendations

A lactation history and observation of a complete breastfeed are fundamental in determining the cause of nipple pain or trauma. The infant's sucking pattern must also be assessed to exclude tongue-tie or any other anomalies. Correct positioning and attachment must be maintained throughout the feed. The mother can be advised to position and feed the infant with the wound at the corner of the infant's mouth to avoid pressure. If the infant is incorrectly attached, the vacuum seal should be released by the mother inserting her clean finger into the corner of the infant's mouth with a little downward pressure. Pulling the infant from the breast without releasing the vacuum will cause further trauma to the nipple. If the nipple is too painful to feed, advise the mother to express breastmilk from the affected side and offer the other breast until she can resume breastfeeding from both sides.

The following treatments may be helpful for cracked nipples; however, as discussed earlier, good quality evidence is limited to support them:

- Expressing breastmilk on to the nipple and rubbing it in following a feed. It is thought the anti-infective properties help protect from infection, although evidence is limited in this area (BFN, 2002).
- Air dry the nipples but avoid rapid drying with the use of hairdryers as this will cause further cracking of the skin.
- Moist wound healing for cracked nipples (BFN, 2002; Lawrence and Lawrence, 2005). Moist wound healing reduces drying of the wound and scab formation by increasing the moisture content of the skin. This can be

in the form of purified lanolin ointment (Lansinoh®) or soft paraffin (for example, Vasoline®) applied sparingly to the nipple following feeding, or the use of various hydrogel wound dressings (such as Jelonet®) (BFN, 2002). When used sparingly, they do not have to be removed before the next feed (Jones, 2008).

Bacterial infection may occur if there is a break in the skin. Infection will lead to delayed wound healing and will need treatment with antibiotics. Common infections include *staphylococcus aureus, escherichia coli* and rarely *streptococcus* (Lawrence and Lawrence, 2005). Mothers may complain of deep breast pain and this must not be confused with thrush.

White spot

The mother may present with a 'white spot' on the nipple and will usually complain of severe 'pin-point' breast pain. On observation of the breast a white spot can be seen on the nipple at the point of the blockage. It is thought to be an overgrowth of epithelium or build-up of fatty material (Spencer, 2008). It can be removed by gentle rubbing or piercing with a sterile needle.

Inverted nipples

Inverted or 'flat' nipples should not affect breastfeeding because, with correct positioning and attachment, the infant latches on to the breast not the nipple. However, many mothers do find inverted or flat nipples a challenge, as do midwives and health visitors when trying to support and advise them. It is important to reassure these mothers that it is possible to successfully breast-feed with inverted nipples, but they may require additional support. Both and Frischnect (2008) recommend the pinch test to see if nipples are truly inverted, by squeezing the areola 2.5cm behind the nipple. If it protrudes it is not a true inverted nipple. Walker (2010, p. 522) describes inverted nipples as follows:

- **Grade I**   There is minimal fibrosis and the nipple can be easily pulled out and maintain protrusion.
- **Grade II**   There is moderate fibrosis beneath the nipple. It can be pulled out but retracts into the areola.
- **Grade III** There are severe fibrotic bands and it is difficult to pull out the nipple.

Practice recommendations

There is no evidence to suggest that antenatal preparation of the nipples is effective in bringing out the nipple (Renfrew *et al.*, 2000), but following the birth there are a number of practices that may help mothers with inverted nipples successfully breastfeed. First, it is important to promote confidence and reassurance that the mother can breastfeed and prolonged skin-to-skin contact will encourage breastfeeding behaviour in both mother and infant (Moore *et al.*, 2009). While establishing breastfeeding she may need to express milk to ensure an adequate milk supply. If the breast is full and taut, and the infant is having difficulty taking the breast into its mouth, it may be helpful to hand express a small amount of milk to soften the breast. There are other techniques that may also help to protrude the nipple (Lawrence and Lawrence, 2005; Walker, 2010), such as:

- Encourage skin-to-skin contact.
- Teach the mother to pull out the nipple and gently roll it before feeds, or to place it between the thumb and the index finger and push backwards to help it protrude.
- Use a breastmilk pump or 'nipplette' prior to breastfeeding to bring out the nipple, to enable the infant to latch on to the breast more effectively.
- Assess for correct positioning and attachment. Suggest positions that aid gravity to enable the infant to scoop a mouthful of breast. If the mother is sat upright or flat this will not help the protrusion of the nipples.
- As a last resort, some mothers may need to use nipple shields during the feed as a temporary measure.

Breast engorgement

Engorgement of the breasts is most often associated with delayed or infrequent feeding, or ineffective removal of the breastmilk. Engorgement is often confused with breast fullness, which occurs in the early days due to increased prolactin levels, increased blood flow to the breast and an increase in milk volume (Smith, 2002).

The engorgement can extend from the breast to include the areola and nipple, and sometimes the mother may experience a low-grade pyrexia. The mother may also complain of pain, particularly before a feed and during the night.

TABLE 5.1 The difference between breast fullness and engorgement

Breast fullness (normal)	Engorgement (not normal)
Warm	Hot
Tender	Painful
Full	Full
Skin: possible marbling	Shiny, possibly inflamed
Milk flows	Milk does not flow easily

Engorgement involves:

- congestion and increased vascularity;
- accumulation of milk;
- oedema (Lawrence and Lawrence, 2005).

If engorgement is not resolved and the milk storage capacity of the breast is exceeded, it can cause the over-distension of the milk-secreting cells, altering their shape, which will decrease further milk production. If there is a build-up of breastmilk and the FIL, this will also contribute to a decrease in milk production (Czank et al., 2007) (see Chapter 2). The congestion can also inhibit lymphatic drainage of toxins and bacteria and predispose the mother to mastitis.

Practice recommendations

A mother with engorgement should be encouraged and supported to empty her breasts regularly (UNICEF, 2008a). This may mean mother-led feeding rather than baby-led or demand feeding. It is crucial at this point to observe a feed to ensure attachment is correct to prevent a decrease in milk production. If the infant is having difficulty attaching to the breast due to the fullness, it can be helpful to express a small amount of breastmilk to make the areola softer, which will make it easier for the infant to attach to the breast.

The pain of engorgement can be quite distressing for mothers. Mangesi and Dowswell (2010) conducted a systematic review to identify treatments for breast engorgement. They examined trials involving acupuncture, cabbage leaves, cold packs, pharmacological treatments and ultrasound, but unfortunately found insufficient evidence to support any of the interventions.

Chilled savoy cabbage leaves are commonly recommended to sooth breast pain. The leaf is placed inside the bra over the breast for 10–15 minutes. Renfrew *et al.* (2005) reviewed two small trials and suggest that cabbage leaves are effective in reducing breast pain caused by engorgement, but it is inconclusive as to whether they should be chilled or not. A warm compress prior to a feed and cold compresses following the feed may be helpful; however, some mothers will require oral analgesia such as paracetamol or ibuprofen.

Blocked ducts

Blocked ducts are usually caused by ineffective removal of breastmilk, resulting in milk stasis in the lactiferous ducts, or by restrictive clothing, such as a tight bra, causing pressure on the outside of the breast (Walker, 2010). Blocked ducts present as localised tenderness and redness in an area of the breast.

Practice recommendations

It is important to observe a complete feed to ensure attachment is correct, otherwise the duct will not be emptied, leading to further discomfort and stasis of the milk, which could develop into mastitis. If breastmilk is not effectively removed there will be a build-up of the FIL and milk production will be reduced. The following measures may be helpful (Walker, 2010):

- Warm compresses prior to a feed, and cold compresses following the feed, may be helpful.
- Massage over the affected area of breast, particularly during a feed, to disperse the blockage.
- During a feed position the infant's chin adjacent to the blocked duct to empty this area of the breast more effectively.
- Avoid constrictive clothing, which may cause stasis of the breastmilk.

Mastitis

Mastitis is the inflammation of the mammary gland. If engorgement or blocked ducts are not corrected and milk stasis persists, it may lead to mastitis and ultimately cessation of breastfeeding. Other causes of mastitis are infrequent or poor emptying of the breast; sore or cracked nipples, which can be a portal for infection; blocked milk ducts; thrush, or candida albicans; and restrictive clothing, such as a tight bra. Frequent breastfeeding can reduce the risk of mothers developing mastitis (Noon, 2010).

Mastitis is usually unilateral, affecting one or two ducts, but can be seen in both breasts. Mastitis is an inflammatory response to breastmilk leaking into the tissue from a blocked duct, and may or may not involve infection (BFN, 2009b). If milk stasis persists and infection ensues it is most commonly due to *staphylococcus aureus* (Walker, 2010).

Mastitis is usually diagnosed clinically and presents with the following symptoms:

- erythema or inflammation of an area of the breast; a hot, red, swollen wedge-shaped area;
- breast pain;
- 'flu-like' symptoms, including fever (temperature in excess of 38.4°C), headache, fatigue and general aches and pains in response to the inflammatory process.

Practice recommendations

- The mother should be encouraged to continue breastfeeding more frequently than usual to ensure the breast is effectively emptied, as not doing so may exacerbate the condition. There is no risk to the infant as mother and infant are colonised with the same organisms. However, some infants appear to dislike the taste of the milk from the affected breast, possibly due to the increased sodium content and, therefore, the milk from this breast may be expressed and discarded. It is crucial to observe a feed to ensure positioning and attachment are correct and that the infant is feeding well.
- Changing positions for feeding may be helpful. Position the infant so that the chin is against the affected part of the breast to assist with drainage.
- Teaching the mother to recognise the signs of an effective feed is essential so that she does not discontinue the feed prematurely (see Chapter 3).
- The mother should also be advised to feed from the affected side first and to express breastmilk at the end of the feed to ensure the breasts are kept as empty as possible, because, on average, infants only fully empty the breast at one or two feeds per day and at most breastfeeds only 67 per cent of the milk available is consumed (Kent, 2007).
- If the mother feels unable to breastfeed she should be encouraged to express regularly. At first, the milk production may be increased; however, the mother should be reassured that this will be temporary and the number of times she expresses can be reduced as the symptoms of mastitis subside.

- Recommend rest and increasing fluid intake.
- A warm compress or shower prior to a feed, and a cold compress following the feed, may be helpful.
- Give non-steroidal anti-inflammatory medications such as ibuprofen 400mgs three times a day (avoid if the mother is asthmatic or has stomach ulcers) and/or paracetamol 1g four times a day to reduce the pyrexia. **Aspirin should not be taken while breastfeeding** (BFN, 2009b).
- Milk culture is rarely used to diagnose infectious mastitis as it is often considered an unreliable test (Spencer, 2008). However, if the problem persists after continued effective removal of breastmilk and approximately two days of antibiotics, milk cultures may be considered.
- Antibiotics are required if the mastitis is thought to be due to infection, usually flucloxacillin 500mgs or erythromycin 500mgs four times a day for ten days (BFN, 2009b). Mothers must be informed that antibiotics may cause the infant to have a loose stool and they must also be vigilant for thrush. Spencer (2008) points out that mastitis resembles inflammatory breast cancer and, when mastitis does not respond to treatment as expected, this should be considered.

Collecting a specimen of breastmilk

If a specimen of breastmilk for culture is required, the correct technique for taking it should be explained to the mothers. She should wash her hands and clean her breast before expressing a small amount of breastmilk. This should then be discarded. She should then express some more breastmilk into a sterile container, avoiding contact with the nipple and container.

Abscesses

An abscess can be a result of mastitis caused by *staphylococcus aureus* and will need to be drained surgically, followed by antibiotics. An abscess can be diagnosed by ultrasound, appearing as a fluid-filled sac (Walker, 2010). Breastfeeding can continue if the mother is well enough, otherwise breastmilk must be expressed to avoid a build-up of FIL.

Preventing the development of a breast abscess

- Effective milk removal and avoidance of milk stasis.
- Treatment of breast inflammation and infection.
- Maternal education regarding position and attachment, demand feeding and avoidance of abrupt weaning.

Thrush or candida albicans

Thrush is rare in the first few weeks of lactation unless the mother has experienced vaginal thrush around the time of the birth (BFN, 2008). It can also occur if either the mother or infant has taken antibiotics or there has been trauma to the nipple.

Diagnosing thrush can be very difficult so, before commencing treatment, other causes for the breast pain must be excluded, such as poor positioning and attachment of the infant to the breast, eczema, tongue-tie, white spot, Raynaud's syndrome or infection.

Signs and symptoms in the mother

- Thrush is usually very painful. The mother often complains of a shooting pain through the breast, which begins during the breastfeed and continues for up to an hour after feeding.
- Initially, breast pain may be localised to one breast but quickly transfers to both.
- The nipple may be red, itchy or sensitive, or have a permanent loss of colour to the nipple and areola. Care must be taken not to confuse this with the temporary loss of colour caused by poor positioning and attachment or Raynaud's syndrome (poor circulation).
- There may be a delay in the healing of cracked nipples.

Signs and symptoms in the infant

- The infant may also exhibit signs of oral thrush (white plaques on the tongue that do not rub away) or nappy rash.
- The infant may keep pulling off the breast, possibly due to a sore mouth or poor attachment, and may be windy and unsettled after a breastfeed.

Practice recommendations

A full lactation history and observation of a feed are essential to rule out problems other than thrush before prescribing medication. The Breastfeeding Network (Jones, 2009b) discourages the use of medication until positioning and attachment have been observed by a skilled practitioner. Mothers should be encouraged to continue feeding to avoid a build-up of the FIL and milk stasis. If they have any frozen breastmilk, it may be best to discard this to prevent reinfection.

If poor positioning and attachment and other causes of breast pain are excluded, both the mother and infant require treatment with antifungal agents:

- **Mother**: Miconazole 2% gel on the nipple and areola. If the nipple is very inflamed, miconazole 2% gel plus 1% hydrocortisone cream. If symptoms persist oral treatment may be required. Fluconazole 150–300mgs loading dose followed by 50–100mgs twice a day is recommended but not licensed for use in lactating women (BFN, 2009c).
- **Infant**: Miconazole gel applied inside the mouth four times a day. However, miconazole is not recommended for infants under four months of age due to the risk of choking; nystatin suspension drops are an alternative (BFN, 2009c).

Up-to-date information for medical treatment is available from www.breast feedingnetwork.org.uk/thrush-and-breastfeeding.html.

Symptoms should subside in two or three days, but if they have not resolved within seven days the general practitioner should be informed.

Mothers should also be advised of other measures that can be helpful (BFN, 2009c), such as:

- Following a feed the breast should be gently rinsed with clear water to remove milk residue.
- Hands should be washed before a breastfeed and following nappy changes.
- Analgesia should be administered, such as paracetamol and ibuprofen.
- Each member of the family should use a separate towel as it can be passed between family members.
- Any dummies, teats and nipple shields should be sterilised, preferably by boiling for 20 minutes, as they are a common cause of reinfection.
- Probiotics may be helpful as well as reducing the level of yeast and sugar in the diet.

Breast refusal

Breast refusal can be very distressing for mothers and undermine their confidence in their ability to breastfeed. Many mothers report feeling that they take it personally and think the infant may not like them. Infants who refuse to breastfeed may exhibit the following signs:

- arching of the back;
- stiffening of the body when approaching the breast;

- pushing the breast away with arms and legs;
- crying;
- extending and turning the head away from the breast.

Breast refusal is commonly associated with an unpleasant event involving breastfeeding, such as someone pushing the head to the breast to encourage feeding. Some mothers report the infant biting them and their startled reaction leading to breast refusal. Other causes may be due to smell, such as changed perfume, washing powder or soap, or the taste of the milk due to a change in diet or medication, or sometimes the onset of menstruation. There may also be issues with the infant, such as teething, ear or nasal obstruction, thrush or other infection.

Other issues must be excluded, such as birth injury resulting in pain or intracranial haemorrhage, oral aversion following suction at birth or other stimulation, hyperlactation or over-active let-down reflex, insufficient milk supply, nipple–teat confusion, or maternal drug abuse or developing illness.

Practice recommendations

Where there is breast refusal it is important not to further exacerbate the problem. The aim is to create a relaxed mother–infant dyad by encouraging a calm and relaxing environment.

- Maximise skin-to-skin opportunities, not only at feeding times, and recommend co-bathing.
- Closely observe for feeding cues and initiate a breastfeed before the infant cries.
- If the infant protests (arching of back, pulling away, crying), discontinue the feeding attempt and calm the infant down. Try again once the infant is calm and displaying feeding cues. There is no point in attempting to put the infant to the breast if it is distressed.
- If the infant does not breastfeed, express breastmilk and give this via a cup or syringe, but try to put the infant to the breast at each feed attempt as described above.
- Breastfeed in a relaxed and quiet environment with no interruptions.
- Advice between professionals must be consistent and therefore a care plan is advisable.

The reluctant feeder or 'sleepy' infant

In the first couple of days following birth infants may feed infrequently, appear sleepy and may not demonstrate feeding cues. Sometimes, even if the infant does latch on to the breast, it may only take a few sucks and fall asleep. This can be a very frustrating problem for mothers and midwives; however, it must be remembered that normal healthy term infants are not at risk because they are able to mobilise glycogen and ketones for energy. Despite this, it is important for the mother to encourage the infant to breastfeed in order to promote the production of prolactin. If the infant does not suckle the mother should hand express at regular intervals.

Some of the reasons for a sleepy infant are:

• maternal analgesia in childbirth;
• birth complications that lead to increased levels of endorphins;
• congenital anomalies or illness;
• birth trauma;
• operative delivery;
• hyperbilirubinaemia (jaundice) and phototherapy;
• prematurity.

Practice recommendations

Mothers can become very upset and express concerns about their ability to breastfeed, so it is extremely important to reassure a mother and teach her techniques that will encourage the infant to feed and also encourage milk production. The midwife should regularly assess the feeds and observe the infant to exclude any signs of illness.

• Encourage undisturbed skin-to-skin contact.
• Encourage uninterrupted access to the breast.
• Attempt to put the infant regularly to the breast followed by hand expression of breastmilk, which can then be given to the infant by cup or syringe.
• Reinforce how to recognise feeding cues.
• Ensure the infant is not too hot or cold when feeding.
• If required, use breast compression to encourage the flow of milk. Place the thumb on the upper side of the breast and the other fingers underneath the breast close to the chest wall. Squeeze, hold and release to increase the internal pressure in the breast to release milk.
• 'Switch' feeding may keep the infant awake (changing from one breast to the other several times during a feed).

This problem usually resolves itself within 36–48 hours, when infants will normally breast 8–12 times a day. If the infant is still sleepy, referral to a paediatrician will be required to exclude underlying illness.

Concluding comments

Many of the common problems of breastfeeding stem from poor positioning and attachment and it is therefore crucial that mothers are taught how to do this correctly and how to recognise an effective breastfeed. The BFI (UNICEF, 2010e) recommends that this is done both verbally and in writing before discharge home. It also advises that a breastfeeding assessment be carried out on the fifth day after birth.

The key areas to remember when addressing breastfeeding problems are:

✔ Take a lactation history.
✔ Observe a complete breastfeed for effective milk transfer, correct position and attachment and sucking pattern.
✔ Observe for breast or nipple anomalies.
✔ Assess the infant's mouth for tongue-tie or any other anomaly.
✔ Encourage skin-to-skin contact.
✔ Use positive language to promote confidence.
✔ Produce a care plan to avoid conflicting advice.

The following chapters, 6 and 7, will explore more specific issues where the mother or infant have special needs that require more specialist advice.

Scenarios

How would you manage the following situations and what advice would you give?

1   On the fifth postnatal day, Carmel tells you she has a cracked right nipple and it is very painful when feeding. She has stopped feeding from that side to let it heal.

2   Alison gave birth to Eve six days ago following a traumatic forceps delivery and postpartum haemorrhage of 1,000ml. When you visit, Alison tells you that Eve is not settling and she does not think she has enough breastmilk and is thinking about changing to formula.

3   Bridget's partner phones you to ask you to visit because Bridget is unwell and has a very painful, red left breast that is hot to the touch. When you arrive she has flu-like symptoms and is in a lot of pain. She has been reluctant to take any medication because she is breastfeeding.

Resources

*   Breastfeeding Network (BFN)
        www.breastfeedingnetwork.org.uk
*   Cochrane Library
        www.thecochranelibrary.com
*   La Leche League
        www.laleche.org.uk

Chapter 6 **Supporting mothers with special needs**

- Learning outcomes
- Human immunodeficiency virus (HIV)
- Herpes simplex virus type 1 (HSV-1)
- Hepatitis B
- Hepatitis C
- Tuberculosis
- Substance misuse
- Delayed lactogenesis
- Caesarean section
- Diabetes
- Obesity
- Polycystic ovary syndrome (PCOS)
- Postpartum haemorrhage
- Breast surgery and anomalies
- Epilepsy
- Hyperlactation or galactorrhea
- Twins
- Concluding comments
- Scenario
- Further reading
- Resources

Most mothers have the ability to breastfeed successfully for the first six months following birth and to continue beyond this, alongside solid food, up to two years and beyond, as recommended by the WHO (2002) and the Department of Health (DH, 2003). However, a small number of mothers may be unable to breastfeed or may have difficulty initiating and maintaining lactation and will require a great deal of support and advice from midwives and health visitors; some may temporarily need to supplement breastfeeding or use breastmilk substitutes. The WHO and UNICEF UK BFI (2009, pp. 8–9) published an updated list of acceptable medical reasons for temporary or long-term use of breastmilk substitutes:

- **Maternal conditions that may justify permanent avoidance of breast-feeding**:
  - HIV infection, if replacement feeding is acceptable, feasible, affordable, sustainable and safe.

- **Maternal conditions that may justify temporary avoidance of breastfeeding**:
  - Severe illness that prevents a mother from caring for her infant, for example sepsis.
  - Herpes simplex virus type 1 (HSV-1).
  - Maternal medication:
    - Sedating psychotherapeutic drugs, anti-epileptic drugs and opioids may cause side effects such as drowsiness and respiratory depression and are better avoided if a safer alternative is available.
    - Radioactive iodine-131 is better avoided. Breastfeeding can resume two months after receiving this substance.
    - Excessive topical iodine or idophors as they can result in thyroid suppression and electrolyte abnormalities.
    - Cytotoxic chemotherapy.

- **Maternal conditions during which breastfeeding can still continue, although health problems may be of concern**:
  - Breast abscess: breastfeeding can continue on the unaffected side and resume on the affected side once treatment has commenced; however, milk must be expressed to prevent exacerbation of the condition (see Chapter 5).
  - Mastitis can be very painful; however, milk must be expressed to prevent exacerbation of the condition (see Chapter 5).
  - Hepatitis B.
  - Tuberculosis.
  - Substance use: mothers should be encouraged to avoid the following and given support and advice to abstain:
    - Nicotine, alcohol, ecstasy, amphetamines, cocaine and other stimulants have demonstrated harmful effects.
    - Alcohol, opioids, benzodiazepines and cannabis can cause sedation in both mother and infant.

This chapter will focus on the issues related to mothers with special needs and some other conditions or situations that may also pose problems and challenges with breastfeeding; Chapter 7 will discuss issues related to infants with special needs.

Learning outcomes

By the end of this chapter you will be able to:

- describe the advice that should be given to HIV-positive mothers in the UK;
- identify those conditions or situations where breastfeeding may be temporarily challenged;
- provide evidence-based information for mothers to help them maintain lactation.

Mapping the UNICEF UK BFI educational outcomes

8   Be equipped to provide parents with accurate, evidence-based information about activities which may have an impact on breastfeeding.

9   Understand the importance of exclusive breastfeeding for the first six months of life and possess the knowledge and skills to enable mothers to achieve this.

16 Understand the limited number of situations in which exclusive breastfeeding is not possible and be able to support mothers in partial breastfeeding or artificial feeding in these circumstances.

Human immunodeficiency virus (HIV)

It is the role of the healthcare professional to provide HIV-positive mothers with information so that they can make an informed choice regarding infant feeding. Therefore, all mothers should be offered an HIV test as part of the antenatal care programme, as well as information about HIV during pregnancy and the implications for the infant. The most common way children are infected by HIV is through vertical transmission before, during or after birth when breastfeeding. This risk is reduced to approximately 2 per cent from up to 45 per cent by treatment with antiretroviral (ARV) drugs, delivery by Caesarean section and avoiding breastfeeding (DH, 2004c). If the mother becomes infected with HIV during breastfeeding, the risk of vertical transmission is greater due to the high viral load than if she was previously infected. Therefore, mothers at risk of acquiring HIV should receive advice on reducing the risk.

Following a systematic review, Horvath *et al.* (2009) recommend complete avoidance of breastfeeding for HIV-positive mothers where possible. However, where this is not possible they recommend two interventions: first, exclusive breastfeeding for the first few months of life; and, second, treating the infant with antiretroviral drugs. Transmission of HIV is more likely if mothers mix-feed (formula and breastfeed) and also if they have mastitis or cracked nipples (Spencer, 2008). Breastfeeding mothers should be taught how to avoid developing mastitis and cracked nipples, but if they do occur they should not breastfeed from the affected breast and instead regularly express breastmilk, ensuring the breast is effectively emptied to prevent cessation of milk production.

The DH (2004c) recognises that breastfeeding is the ideal way to feed infants; however, it does highlight that it is a route for mother–child (vertical) transmission and recommends the 'avoidance of all breastfeeding by HIV-infected women' (DH, 2004c, p. 2). The DH recommendation relates only to the UK and does not include less developed countries. The WHO (2010b) also recommends that HIV-infected mothers should not breastfeed if replacement feeding is acceptable in the society and if parents can afford formula and sustain it for six months, which includes having access to appropriate facilities to prepare formula safely, in hygienic conditions, with safe water. Where this is not possible, the WHO (2010b) now recommends that exclusive breastfeeding should continue for six months and can continue until 12 months of age alongside the introduction of other foods, provided the mother and/or infant continue to take the antiretroviral drugs, which they suggest the mother should commence at 14 weeks' gestation. Evidence demonstrates that, with strict adherence to the antiretroviral regime in pregnancy and during breastfeeding, the HIV infection rate may be as low as 2 per cent (WHO, 2010b). Unfortunately, some mothers and infants will not have access to these medications and the advice for them remains the same as previously (see Table 6.1). Mothers in this category are advised to breastfeed exclusively for no more than the first six months of life and then abruptly wean, introducing a breastmilk substitute along with solid foods.

The issue of infant feeding should be raised as early as possible with HIV-positive mothers, or those at risk, and it will be the mother's informed decision how she intends to feed. Either way, parents will need support and advice: for breastfeeding mothers, how to avoid the risks of vertical transmission; and for those who choose to formula feed how to safely make up a feed and sterilise equipment.

TABLE 6.1 Changes to the WHO infant feeding guidelines for HIV-positive mothers

2006 WHO guidelines	2010 WHO guidelines
Mother: take ARVs from 28 weeks' gestation	Mother: take ARVs from 14 weeks' gestation
Short ARV regime during breastfeeding period for mother and/or infant	Long ARV regime during breastfeeding period for mother and/or infant
Exclusive breastfeeding for 6 months	Exclusive breastfeeding for 6 months
Abrupt weaning from breastmilk	Gradually wean from the breast but continue for the first 12 months of life; only stop when an adequate and safe diet without breastmilk is available
	Gradually stop breastfeeding within 1 month but continue ARVs for 1 week
	Avoid abrupt weaning
No mixed feeding	Complementary feed after 6 months
Not recommended to breastfeed after 6 months	Recommend to breastfeed or mix-feed in conjunction with ARVs

Source: adapted from WHO (2010b).

HIV is the only indication highlighted by the DH (2003b), where breast-feeding is not recommended. The rest of this chapter will focus on situations in which breastfeeding is challenging.

Herpes simplex virus type 1 (HSV-1)

HSV-1 is the virus that normally causes cold sores around the mouth but in the newborn can affect the immune system. Although HSV-1 can be found in the breastmilk of symptomatic mothers there is no evidence to suggest vertical transmission is a problem. However, HSV-1 can be transmitted by direct contact (Sullivan-Boylai *et al.*, 2001) and therefore direct contact between the lesions on the mother's breasts or mouth and the infant should be avoided. This may have implications for skin-to-skin contact. If the lesions are on the breast, feeding from that side should be avoided until it has cleared up. Nevertheless, the breast must be regularly emptied by expression to avoid a build-up of FIL and to maintain the milk supply in the affected breast; the expressed milk should be discarded. Feeding from the unaffected side can continue as normal. Antiviral drugs such as acyclovir can be prescribed and are safe during breastfeeding (Jones, 2009a). Mothers should also be educated about the importance of hand washing, washing of blankets and towels and avoiding kissing the infant if the lesions are on the mouth.

Hepatitis B

Hepatitis B is a serious liver infection that can cause liver failure or cirrhosis. It is transmitted via infected blood and other body fluids. In 2000, the DH recommended that all pregnant women should be offered screening. Infants of those mothers who test positive for hepatitis B should be given hepatitis B vaccine and hepatitis B immune globulin (HBIG) as soon as possible, preferably within the first 12 hours of life. This will give a 95 per cent protection rate for the infant. Additional doses to complete the treatment will be administered at one and six months of age. Without this treatment there is a 90 per cent risk of infection (DH, 2000; Hepatitis B Foundation, 2007). Preterm infants weighing less than 2,000g at birth should be vaccinated at one month of age. The DH (2000, 2007b) and the Hepatitis B Foundation (2009) recommend breastfeeding for infants who are immunised as the benefits outweigh the potential risk of infection.

Hepatitis C

Hepatitis C is a disease of the liver caused by the hepatitis C virus (HCV), which may develop into cirrhosis of the liver, liver failure or liver cancer. There is no vaccine for HCV. It is a blood-borne virus that is not transmitted in breastmilk and therefore mothers should be advised to breastfeed (Scottish Government, 2002).

Tuberculosis

Mothers at risk of tuberculosis (TB) are those who have been in an area where it is endemic or in close contact with someone who has the active disease. Women who are HIV positive or are immunosuppressed are also at risk. The risk to the fetus in utero is minimal and, if treated, prognosis is good. However, if untreated, the newborn can become infected through close contact with its mother. Screening for TB should be offered to those at risk (for example, through recent exposure to TB, or HIV positive).

TB is not transmitted through breastmilk. Mothers infected with TB and taking treatment can breastfeed because the concentrations of the medication in breastmilk are too small to be toxic. Mothers taking isoniazid should also take 10–25mg pyridoxine (vitamin B6) supplementation daily (Health Protection Agency, 2006).

Substance misuse

Substance misuse and breastfeeding is a contentious issue and healthcare professionals need to weigh up the risk/benefit ratio when advising mothers about the benefits of breastfeeding; however, this may be difficult because there is limited research in this area. Most drugs will be transferred to the infant through breastmilk, but most are at such low levels that they will not cause harm to the breastfeeding infant (Hale *et al.*, 2007). McCrory (2007, p. 206) describes it as a 'theoretical situation'; because the infant is getting some of the drug it could be considered unadvisable, but in reality the fetus is getting larger amounts in utero. These infants are vulnerable and are at higher risk of SIDS, poor nutrition and weight gain due to the chaotic lifestyle their mothers often lead; therefore the benefits of breastfeeding may outweigh the negative effects of the drug abuse and lifestyle. The exceptions to this advice are for mothers taking large amounts of cocaine, amphetamines/metamphetamine, or benzo-diazepines, where breastfeeding is contraindicated (WA Centre for Evidence Based Nursing & Midwifery, 2007; McAfee, 2007). Cannabis use is thought to suppress the production of prolactin and, additionally, causes many of the problems associated with smoking because it is usually combined with tobacco; it is therefore advisable to avoid breastfeeding for several hours after smoking cannabis (Amir, 2002; McAfee, 2007). Effects on the infant are unclear, but it is thought to cause drowsiness, poor feeding and developmental delay.

Dryden *et al.* (2009) conducted a retrospective cohort study of 450 drug-dependent women from an inner-city hospital to investigate factors associated with the development of neonatal abstinence syndrome (NAS) and the implications for healthcare resources. They found that infants who were breastfed for more than 72 hours were less likely to require treatment for NAS. They suggested this could be due to the benefits of breastmilk combined with the small traces of drug in the breastmilk lessening withdrawal symptoms, and the soothing effect of breastfeeding. They recommend these mothers should have an increased length of postnatal stay in hospital and increased support to continue breastfeeding while observing for signs of NAS in the infant. Jambert-Gray *et al.* (2009) support these findings and highlight the importance of breastfeeding to improving self-esteem and suggest that these mothers may be more likely to wean themselves off methadone.

Smoking

Although smoking while breastfeeding is not recommended, the benefits of breastmilk outweigh the risks from nicotine. Dorea states that it is 'worse to smoke and not breastfeed' (2007, p. 290). Nicotine is found in breastmilk and

Practice recommendations

- Avoid separation; if treatment for NAS is required this can be done on the postnatal ward.
- Prolong skin-to-skin contact to encourage breastfeeding and bonding, regulate the infant's heart and respiratory rate and temperature, reduce crying and sooth irritability.
- If there is separation encourage regular expression of breastmilk.

To minimise harm:
- Discourage injection of drugs because of the risk of transmitting HIV.
- Breastfeed immediately before drug use.
- Express before drug use so that breastmilk is available.
- Monitor the infant for signs of NAS.
- Do not sleep with the infant in bed or on the settee.

Further information on specific drugs can be found in Hale, T. (2008) *Medications and Mothers Milk*, Amarillo, TX: Pharmasoft Medical Publishing, and Hale, T. and Hartmann, P. (eds) (2007) *Textbook of Human Lactation*, Amarillo, TX: Hale Publishing.

will alter the taste. Mothers who smoke have a reduced milk supply and have a shorter duration of breastfeeding than their counterparts (Amir, 2002). It is proposed that nicotine inhibits the production of prolactin; however, further research is required in this area. Excessive crying, fussiness and colic in infants of mothers who smoke are reported, which may lead to cessation of breast-feeding because of the mothers' perception of insufficient milk supply (Giglia *et al.*, 2006). Infants also sleep less after breastfeeding when their mothers have smoked before the feed (Mannella *et al.*, 2007).

During pregnancy all mothers who smoke should be offered support and help to stop smoking and, where available, referral to a smoking cessation practitioner who will provide advice on how to give up or reduce smoking. Nicotine replacement therapy is thought to decrease the amount of nicotine transferred in breastmilk. If the mother chooses to continue to smoke while breastfeeding, she should be advised not to smoke before a feed but after-wards, because it takes approximately 95 minutes for nicotine to be cleared from breastmilk, with levels peaking 30–60 minutes after smoking a cigarette (Jones, 2009b). She should also be encouraged to smoke away from the infant as passive smoking is also a risk factor for SIDS, respiratory infections and asthma.

Alcohol

In recent years, recommendations about alcohol consumption while breast-feeding have been confusing for mothers and professionals alike because of a lack of robust research. Alcohol does pass into breastmilk and will affect the smell and taste. Current guidelines suggest that drinking one or two units of alcohol once or twice a week is not harmful while breastfeeding, but more than this may interfere with the let-down reflex (DH, 2006; NHS Choices, 2009) and potentially affect the infant's development. In the past, mothers were erroneously advised to drink alcohol to increase their milk production. This may have been because alcohol can increase prolactin levels immediately, but after an hour of consumption the levels are decreased, as is milk yield (Menella and Pepino, 2008). It also has a negative effect on oxytocin and milk ejection. Milk volume is reduced by 23 per cent after one alcoholic unit (Fisher, 1998). Because of the lack of conclusive research many mothers may choose not to drink alcohol at all while breastfeeding.

However, if a mother chooses to drink alcohol it should be avoided before a feed, as it takes approximately two hours to clear alcohol from the breastmilk and peak levels appear at approximately 30–90 minutes following intake (Giglia and Binns, 2008). As feeding is unpredictable, some mothers choose to plan when they are going to consume alcohol and express milk to feed their infant.

Key fact

Breastfeeding mothers can eat peanuts while breastfeeding as part of a healthy balanced diet, unless they are allergic to them (DH, 2009a).

Delayed lactogenesis

Lactogenesis II is the onset of milk production and occurs following expulsion of the placenta and membranes, which results in a sudden drop in progesterone and oestrogen levels (neuroendocrine control). As prolactin levels increase, it binds with prolactin receptors in the walls of the lactocytes and begins milk synthesis (Lawrence and Lawrence, 2005). Skin-to-skin contact at birth with the infant stimulates the production of prolactin and oxytocin. Early and regular breastfeeding inhibits the production of the prolactin-inhibiting factor (PIF) and stimulates production of prolactin. Lactogenesis II commences 30–40 hours after birth, but mothers do not feel the milk 'coming in' until about 2–3 days after birth (see Chapter 2).

Lactogenesis III is the autocrine regulation where supply and demand regulate milk production. A whey protein called the feedback inhibitor of lactation (FIL) is secreted by the lactocytes. As the alveoli distend there is a build-up of FIL and milk synthesis is inhibited. When the breastmilk is effectively removed and the concentrations of FIL reduce, milk synthesis resumes. This is a local mechanism and can occur in one or both breasts. It exerts a negative feedback response to inhibit milk production when there is ineffective removal of the breastmilk from the breast (see Chapter 2).

Mothers who experience delayed onset of lactogenesis II are more likely to have shorter duration of breastfeeding and therefore need a lot of support and encouragement. The most common reason for delayed lactogenesis II is ineffective removal of milk from the breast, usually due to poor position and attachment or delayed suckling. However, there may be certain factors that inhibit effective removal of breastmilk or influence delay of lactogenesis II such as:

- Breast surgery
- Obesity
- Diabetes
- Retained products of conception
- Polycystic ovaries
- Caesarean section
- Anxiety and lack of confidence
- Preterm birth
- Hormonal problems
 (Dewey *et al.*, 2005)

Some of these factors will be discussed further in this chapter and in Chapter 7, but the plan of care for any condition or problem that may result in delayed lactogenesis should follow the same main principles to encourage lactation:

- skin-to-skin contact;
- early and regular feeding or expression;
- avoiding separation of mother and infant where possible;
- regular assessment of milk transfer.

Caesarean section

Following Caesarean section mothers are at risk of delayed lactation (Rowe-Murray and Fisher, 2002). Baxter (2006) conducted a quantitative survey of 422 women in England who had given birth by Caesarean section, with a 65 per cent response rate, to explore their experiences of breastfeeding. She found that 84 per cent of the sample commenced breastfeeding, of which 65 per cent were still breastfeeding between five and eight weeks after giving birth. The most common reason for giving up breastfeeding was the perception of insufficient milk and inconvenience. Other reasons cited were lack of support, difficulty with attachment and pain.

Key fact

Caffeine is transferred in breastmilk and may keep the infant awake and cause irritability. It is therefore advisable to avoid drinks containing caffeine where possible (DH, 2009a) or have a maximum of 2–3 cups of coffee per day after feeds. Caffeine levels peak one hour after consumption. Iron levels in breastmilk are reduced when drinking more than three cups of coffee a day.

Hospital practices following a Caesarean section may inhibit lactation. Following a Caesarean section mothers will have intravenous infusions, a catheter and pain from the scar site. Therefore, it is particularly important to assist the mother following Caesarean section in practical issues such as easy access to the infant and ensuring she is in a comfortable position to attach her infant to the breast.

Most Caesarean section incisions are now in the lower segment of the uterus, thus making it difficult to hold the infant in the cradle position. Other suggested positions for breastfeeding are the mother lying on her side, the 'underarm' hold or putting a pillow over her lap to place the baby on to avoid pressure on her scar.

Practice recommendations

- Skin-to-skin contact in theatre if possible and to continue as long as possible. If the mother is unable to provide skin-to-skin contact, the father should be encouraged to do so.
- Early and regular breastfeeding or regular expressing eight to ten times a day to promote lactation. To ensure lactation is adequate there should be careful assessment of the infant's hydration, wet nappies and changing stool, and signs of jaundice.
- If separated, ensure a visit is arranged as soon as possible and encourage expressing in front of the infant to aid the let-down reflex.
- Ensure the environment is conducive to breastfeeding and provide ongoing skilled support, particularly with positioning and attachment.

Diabetes

There are three types of diabetes breastfeeding mothers may have:

- type 1 diabetes (insulin-dependent diabetes – beta cells of the pancreas do not produce insulin);
- type 2 diabetes (non-insulin diabetes – metabolic disorder, associated with obesity, where insulin is present but receptor cells do not respond);
- gestational diabetes (glucose intolerance developed in pregnancy).

Infants born to mothers with diabetes are at greater risk of prematurity, macrosomia, birth by Caesarean section, respiratory problems, congenital abnormalities, hypocalcaemia, polycythaemia and hyperbilirubinaemia (Taylor *et al.*, 2005). Following birth, newborns are also at greater risk of hypoglycaemia because of maternal hyperinsulinism in pregnancy, resulting in neonatal hypoglycaemia. However, Chertok *et al.* (2009) demonstrated higher blood glucose levels in infants that were breastfed within the first 30 minutes of birth compared to those who did not receive an early breast or received artificial milk for the first feed.

Mothers with diabetes have a delay in lactogenesis II of approximately a day, which can result in a reduced milk intake for infants (Hartmann and Cregan, 2001). It is therefore important to avoid separation and to encourage early feeding. If separation is unavoidable, the mother should be encouraged to express frequently, eight to ten times a day. Walker (2010) suggests that a diabetic mother could express colostrum from 34 weeks' pregnancy, freeze it and bring it to hospital in case the newborn baby requires a supplement. She recommends that the mother expresses each breast for three to five minutes and that the colostrum can be collected in a small syringe. However, if the mother experiences uterine tightening she should stop.

Diabetic mothers who choose to breastfeed lose weight more quickly and have also been found to have more stable blood glucose levels, requiring approximately 27 per cent less insulin than their pre-pregnancy requirement. Too much and too little insulin also influences milk production (Alban-Davies *et al.*, 1989).

Approximately 525–625 additional calories per day (total approximately 2,500–2,800 calories per day) are required by the mother during breastfeeding, 200kcal of which is mobilised from fat stores laid down during pregnancy (Jackson, 2004). It is thought that type 1 diabetic mothers may require an additional 50g of carbohydrate per day to ensure adequate lactation. Jackson (2004) recommends that the mother checks her blood glucose before each feed, even at night, and eats a snack to prevent hypoglycaemia. The mother must also be made aware that it is normal to feel more thirsty during breastfeeding, and by checking her blood glucose level she should be able to differentiate this thirst from that of the symptoms of hyperglycaemia.

Practice recommendations

- Skin-to-skin contact. As well as encouraging an early breastfeed, this will reduce crying, regulate temperature and breathing, and thus conserve energy and reduce the risk of hypoglycaemia.
- In response to the delayed lactogenesis, encourage breastfeeding eight to ten times a day or express breastmilk if this is not possible.
- To ensure lactation is adequate, there should be careful assessment of the infant's hydration, wet nappies and changing stool, and signs of jaundice.
- Hypoglycaemia can be a problem for insulin-dependent diabetics. If the mother's blood glucose is low, she should have a high-sugar snack such as a milkshake or biscuit (Jackson, 2004). It is important to avoid a hypo-glycaemic attack when breastfeeding; if it does occur, Jackson (2004) suggests rapid treatment of one of the following: three or four glucose tablets, 150ml lucozade or fruit juice, or 200ml of a fizzy drink followed by a high-carbohydrate food such as bread or cereal.
- If the mother develops cracked nipples, thrush or mastitis, she should treat her diabetes as she would with any other illness and monitor her blood glucose very carefully and alter her insulin as required to avoid hyper-glycaemia (Jackson, 2004).

Obesity

In 2008, 42 per cent of men and 32 per cent of women in England were classified as overweight (body mass index (BMI) $25kg/m^2$ to less than $30kg/m^2$), and 24 per cent of men and 25 per cent of women aged 16 years and over were classified as obese (BMI $30Kg/m^2$ or over) (NHS Information Centre, 2010). Women who are obese are at greater risk of developing conditions that challenge successful breastfeeding, such as diabetes mellitus, gestational diabetes, postpartum haemorrhage and pre-eclampsia. They are also at greater risk of having a Caesarean section, which makes them significantly less likely to breastfeed (Rowe-Murray and Fisher, 2002; Taylor et al., 2005; Rasmussen, 2007). Infants born to obese mothers are also more likely to be post-mature (>42 weeks gestation), have macrosomia and poor APGAR scores, and be admitted to the neonatal unit (Rasmussen, 2007). Higher rates of obstetric and neonatal problems associated with obesity may also lead to separation of the mother and infant.

Women with a BMI greater than $29kg/m^2$ have been associated with delayed lactogenesis II and reduced duration of breastfeeding due to lower levels of prolactin (Rasmussen and Kjolhede, 2004). Rasmussen and Kjolhede (2004) suggest that this may be due to the fact that progesterone is a fat-soluble hormone. In obese women the rate of clearance of progesterone following birth may be delayed, thus inhibiting the action of prolactin on the lactocytes. The delay in lactogenesis II can be as much as 60 hours. Walker (2010) suggests that the problem is exacerbated by the tendency for obese women to have large heavy breasts, large areolas and, often, flat nipples, which may contribute to problems with positioning and attachment, resulting in poor milk supply and nipple trauma.

Practice recommendations

- Skin-to-skin contact.
- Encourage to feed eight to ten times a day until lactogenesis II is established to encourage lactation. Infants of obese mothers have higher levels of plasma insulin and are therefore at risk of hypoglycaemic episodes that could lead to seizures. Regular feeding will alleviate this and avoid the need for supplementation, ensuring the infant is well hydrated and preventing weight loss.
- Avoid maternal–infant separation where possible.
- Positioning the baby at the breast will be a challenge and obese mothers will need a lot of encouragement and support. Large heavy breasts may need support, such as a rolled-up towel under the breast. Care must be taken if the baby is being fed in the underarm position so that the heavy breasts do not lie on top of the baby (Walker, 2010). Ongoing support is required for obese mothers as they are less likely to continue breastfeeding.
- Some obese mothers may feel anxious and embarrassed, which will have a negative effect on the let-down reflex. It is important therefore to provide emotional support and to provide an environment that is conducive to putting the mother at ease.
- If the mother's nipples are flat, she may need to use a syringe or a breast pump first to pull the nipples out (see Chapter 5).
- Careful hygiene of the skin folds of the breasts is important to avoid itching and infection.

There is also confusion as to whether mothers who have had bariatric surgery can breastfeed. Breastfeeding is possible; however, both the mother and baby may need vitamin B12 supplements to avoid complications (Walker, 2010).

Polycystic ovary syndrome (PCOS)

Polycystic ovary syndrome is a complex syndrome causing ovarian, endocrine and metabolic dysfunction. Ovaries are usually bigger than usual with a large number of small follicles on the outer surface that rarely ovulate. Because a woman with PCOS rarely ovulates, fertility is a major problem. Other signs of PCOS may include menstrual disturbances, obesity, acne and hirsutism (excessive body hair), but they may not be present in all women. Those who develop PCOS in adolescence are at higher risk of diabetes and cardiovascular problems (Walker, 2010).

Approximately 10 per cent of the female population is thought to have PCOS, but not all will present with health problems and may not know they have it until they have problems with breastfeeding – usually insufficient milk supply. Marasco and Marmet (2000) suggested that approximately one third of women with PCOS had normal milk supply; however, where there is poor milk supply it may be due to:

- low oestrogen levels resulting in poor mammary development in puberty;
- high levels of androgen hormones that inhibit prolactin working on the receptor sites;
- increased oestrogen levels after birth that interfere with lactation;
- diabetes or obesity.

Some mothers with PCOS may also have an overproduction of milk (galactorrhea – see later in this chapter). Either way, mothers with PCOS need a great deal of support and encouragement to commence breastfeeding and to continue.

Practice recommendations

- Skin-to-skin contact.
- Early and frequent feeding with additional milk expression.
- Galactagogues may be required.
- Close monitoring of milk transfer and that the infant is thriving.

Postpartum haemorrhage

Postpartum haemorrhage can impede lactogenesis II by inhibiting the production of prolactin and, in rare cases, can result in Sheehan's syndrome (necrosis of the pituitary gland) (Willis and Livingstone, 1995). Cortisol levels may also be increased due to the traumatic nature of the labour and add to the adverse affect on lactogenesis (Thompson *et al.*, 2010).

Practice recommendations

- Skin-to-skin contact.
- Early and regular breastfeeding.
- Avoid maternal–infant separation.
- Empty the breast by feeding or expressing as frequently as possible in the first two weeks (approximately eight to ten times a day) to maximise milk production capacity.
- Provide continuing support and education, with position and attachment and assessment of breastfeeds.
- Assess milk transfer by close observation of the baby: weight, and nappies for urine and stool (see Chapter 3).

Early and regular breastfeeding will also stimulate the production of oxytocin, which will cause uterine contraction and reduce blood loss (Thompson *et al.*, 2010).

Breast surgery and anomalies

Breast anomalies can be congenital or acquired, and can cause serious problems for women who would like to breastfeed but, due to the lack of confidence, find it difficult. Ectopic breasts (mammary heterotopia), or supernumerary breast tissue, is the most common congenital abnormality and can be found anywhere on the milk line from the axilla to pubic region, although 20 per cent occur in the axilla and may lactate following childbirth. These women need extra support to increase their confidence and also to teach effective positioning and attachment.

Breast surgery for augmentation or reduction may also pose problems with lactation (Souto *et al.*, 2003). However, increasingly surgeons are developing techniques that preserve the lactiferous ducts, but evidence remains sparse regarding the effect on breastfeeding (Nommsen-Rivers, 2003). The aim of breast reduction is to remove the volume of breast tissue, which includes both glandular and fatty tissue and which may result in reduced milk-producing ability. There are numerous surgical techniques, but it appears that mothers who are more likely to breastfeed successfully have had surgery that does not completely sever the areola and nipple, but instead moves them while still being attached to the 'pedicle', ducts, nerves and blood supply. Many women have reduced nipple sensation following the procedure, which may negatively affect the let-down reflex. Some mothers may also complain of oversensitivity during the healing process. Bearing in mind that some women may only have nine main ducts (Ramsay *et al.*, 2005), removal of any of these is likely to cause a reduction in milk supply.

Breast augmentation is the insertion of either a silicone or saline-filled implant either under the chest wall, where the tissue and nerves are relatively undisturbed, or on top of the muscle next to the glandular tissues, which may cause greater interference with milk production. The techniques used for inserting the implant are:

- *transaxillary*: near the axilla but placed below the muscle;
- *inframammary*: under the breast but placed on top of the muscle next to the glandular tissue, which may cause pressure;
- *transumbilical*: via the umbilicus, placing the implant above the muscle next to the glandular tissue, causing more tissue disruption;
- *periareolar*: incision around the areola resulting in ductal, glandular and nerve damage; the implant is also inserted above the muscle.

Practice recommendations

- Establish a good history regarding the breast problem or type of surgery.
- Skin-to-skin contact.
- Early and regular breastfeeding.
- Avoid maternal–infant separation.
- Empty the breast by feeding or expressing as frequently as possible in the first two weeks (approximately eight to ten times a day) to maximise milk production capacity.
- Provide continuing support with position and attachment and assessment of breastfeeds.
- Assess milk transfer by close observation of the baby: weight, and nappies for urine and stool (see Chapter 3).

Some mothers with breast anomalies, or following breast surgery, report production of colostrum but do not go on to lactate fully. Therefore, careful observation of the infant is required to ensure there is effective milk production and transfer and that the infant is thriving. It must also be remembered that the mother may have had surgery for poorly developed breasts, which may have been a consequence of polycystic ovaries.

Epilepsy

Mothers with epilepsy should be encouraged to breastfeed (SIGN, 2003; NICE, 2004). Small amounts of anti-epileptic drugs (AEDs) pass into the breastmilk; however, the levels of the drugs found in breastmilk are thought to be lower than the fetus is exposed to in utero and therefore not contraindicated in breastfeeding (Walker, 2010). Breastfeeding may therefore reduce withdrawal symptoms in the newborn, such as hyperirritability and poor sucking. However, some drugs may have side effects that may cause the infant to be sleepy and lead to difficulties with maintaining attachment. Mothers will need support to establish lactation and ensure adequate milk transfer. They should feed regularly and may need to express milk as well to ensure an adequate milk supply. It is also important for the mother to consider where she feeds her infant so that, if she does have a seizure, the risk of an accident is minimised. It is advisable to sit on the floor or an area where the infant will not fall.

Hyperlactation or galactorrhea

Hyperlactation is the overproduction of breastmilk and can be caused by breastfeeding mismanagement, medications or hyperprolactinaemia. The mother will have a constant feeling of fullness and may leak or spray copious amounts of milk from the other breast during feeding, and she will leak in between feeds. Because the breasts are always full, she is at higher risk of mastitis and developing an abscess. Livingstone (1996) suggested that problems are most likely to occur when the mother switches her infant from one breast to the other before the first has been effectively emptied and the infant has had a chance to receive the high-fat milk, or because of poor position and attachment.

Hyperlactation may also pose problems for the infant during a feed as it struggles to cope with the flow of the feed, possibly resulting in breast refusal. Also, the infant may be unable to empty the breast adequately to get the high-fat milk, which will result in poor weight gain and failure to thrive. The infant will also present with colic and explosive, watery, green stools (see Figure 6.1).

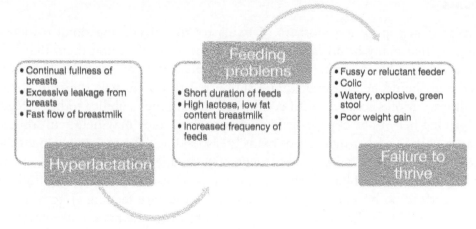

- Continual fullness of breasts
- Excessive leakage from breasts
- Fast flow of breastmilk

Hyperlactation

Feeding problems

- Short duration of feeds
- High lactose, low fat content breastmilk
- Increased frequency of feeds

- Fussy or reluctant feeder
- Colic
- Watery, explosive, green stool
- Poor weight gain

Failure to thrive

FIGURE 6.1 The consequences of hyperlactation

Practice recommendations

There is limited evidence available regarding the management of hyperlactation; however, the aim is to improve milk removal and drainage in each breast. Livingstone (1996) recommends that the way to treat hyperlactation is not by reducing the frequency of breastfeeding, but instead restricting feeds to one breast only to allow a reduction of milk supply to occur through the build-up of the FIL in the other breast. By feeding at one breast only, the infant is more likely to drain the breast effectively, receiving the fattier milk, which will be more satisfying and thus increase time intervals between feeds. However, Livingstone does identify the increased risk of blocked ducts and mastitis, and therefore this management requires careful monitoring.

Another suggestion is *block feeding*, whereby the infant is offered the same breast for a block period of time during the day and will have several consecutive feeds at this breast before doing the same on the other (vanVeldhuizen-Staas, 2007). Van Veldhuizen-Staas (2007) recommends full drainage and block feeding. This starts with, as near as possible, complete drainage of both breasts using a mechanical breast pump. The infant is then offered the breasts where they will receive high-fat milk. She suggests that this may have been the first time these infants will have had high-fat milk and they will be satiated and sleep following the feed. The rest of the day is split into blocks of time starting with three hours. As the infant demands a feed, the same breast is offered for that block of time. At the end of this block of time the infant will be offered the other breast for all the demanded feeds in the next block of time. The time blocks should be individually assessed depending on the individual symptoms.

Herbal remedies are also thought to reduce milk supply, such as sage and peppermint tea (Walker, 2010).

Twins

Rather than supporting mothers of twins to breastfeed, anecdotal evidence suggests that many healthcare professionals are still informing them that it is not possible. This is untrue; mothers of multiple births can successfully breast-feed and should be encouraged and supported to do so. It is the role of the healthcare professional to instil confidence in a mother's ability to breastfeed. Informing her of any support groups during pregnancy may help with this so that she can see other mothers of twins breastfeeding. The main challenges the mother faces are prematurity (see Chapter 7), tiredness and time. Twins can be fed separately or simultaneously; however, it is advisable to encourage mothers to breastfeed both infants together, as soon as they are feeding effectively, to reduce the time feeding takes and also to establish an adequate milk supply.

The most common position for feeding is the underarm hold, but any position the mother can manage that adheres to the principles of positioning and attachment will work. Some mothers find a V-shaped pillow useful to support the infants when feeding them simultaneously in the early days, but care must be taken that it does not interfere with positioning and attachment (see Figure 6.2).

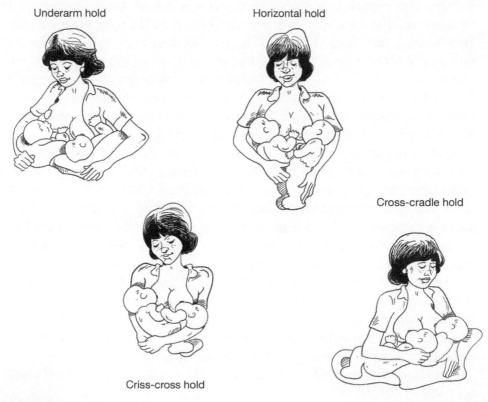

Underarm hold

Horizontal hold

Cross-cradle hold

Criss-cross hold

FIGURE 6.2 Breastfeeding positions with twins

Tiredness is a common complaint and family and friends often ask to help by feeding the twins. It would be more helpful if they helped with family chores such as cooking, cleaning, washing and ironing or looking after other children, to allow the mother time to rest and spend with her twins to establish breastfeeding.

Concluding comments

HIV is the only condition where the DH recommends that breastfeeding should be avoided. However, there are a number of conditions or situations where breastfeeding may need to be temporarily avoided or may compromise the initiation, duration and exclusivity of breastfeeding. This chapter has described some of the situations healthcare professionals may come into contact with in clinical practice, but it is by no means exhaustive.

Although many of these conditions or situations have individual complexities, it is clear that the principles of establishing and maintaining an adequate milk supply are very similar. In all cases it is important that a detailed lactation history is taken, followed by observation of a full breastfeed to observe for position and attachment and milk transfer. Breastfeeding straight after birth is crucial, where possible, followed by regular stimulation of the breast by the infant or expressing by hand or with a pump. Skin-to-skin contact should also be recommended at any age. Ongoing support by knowledgeable healthcare practitioners is essential for mothers in challenging situations.

Scenario

Jonathan is four days old. He was 4kg at birth and had rather a hard entry into the world. After a 14-hour first stage, his mother Anne had pushed for nearly two hours with little progress. After some discussion, Jonathan was delivered using Kielland's rotational forceps. Anne sustained a 1,500ml postpartum haemorrhage, was transfused two units of packed red blood cells and also had a third-degree tear. As Anne was symptomatic post-delivery and had to go to theatre to be sutured, she had consented to Jonathan having a cup feed, as she was unable to feed him initially.

His first breastfeed was when he was ten hours old, although he had a 50ml cup feed two hours after birth and again at eight hours. He had never been skin-to-skin with Anne immediately following birth. Yesterday he weighed 3.7kg and the paediatricians requested that he be weighed again today. Today he is 3.6kg. Anne's breasts are reported as being soft.

- **What would you do?**

Further reading

- WHO (2010) *Guidelines on HIV and Infant Feeding: Principles and Recommendations for Infant Feeding in the Context of HIV and a Summary of Evidence*, Geneva: WHO.
- WHO/UNICEF (2009) *Acceptable Medical Reasons for the Use of Breast-milk Substitutes*, Geneva: WHO.

Resources

- UKMiCentral quick reference guide, *Drugs in Breastmilk*
  www.ukmicentral.nhs.uk
- Twins and Multiple Births Association (TAMBA)
  www.tamba.org.uk
- Multiple Births Foundation
  www.multiplebirths.org.uk

Chapter 7 **Infants with special needs**

Breastmilk should be the first choice of infant nutrition for infants separated from their mothers or for those with special needs. Exclusive breastfeeding should be protected, with no other food or drugs being given, unless medically indicated, because of the benefits breastmilk confers on both mother and infant (WHO, 2002).

Infants with special needs, such as low birthweight and prematurity, are at higher risk of poor outcomes following birth, throughout childhood and on to adulthood. A high proportion of infants from this category are also from disadvantaged socio-economic backgrounds (Moser, Whittle *et al.*, 2003). In neonatal units parents are increasingly encouraged to provide breastmilk for their infants as part of the care package and this presents a great opportunity for healthcare professionals to promote breastfeeding.

There will be situations when breastmilk substitutes will be required; however, these should be medically indicated and clear protocols developed to deal with these situations. The WHO and UNICEF (2009, p. 7) published an updated list of acceptable medical reasons for temporary or long-term use of breastmilk substitutes:

- **Infants who should not receive breastmilk or any other milk except specialised formula:**

  - *Infants with galactosemia*:
    This is a rare genetic trait incompatible with breastfeeding. Symptoms include vomiting, jaundice, hepatosplenomegaly and bleeding. Without treatment galactose builds up and can cause kidney, liver, nerve and eye damage. A special galactose-free formula is needed (Lawrence and Lawrence, 2005).

  - *Infants with maple syrup urine disease*:
    This is an aminoacidopathy and presents with poor feeding and weight gain, vomiting, seizures and lethargy. Breastfeeding may delay onset of these symptoms. Breastfeeding is possible but infants require careful monitoring and supplementation with a special formula free of leucine, isoleucine and valine (Hunter *et al.*, 2005).

  - *Infants with phenylketonuria*:
    A special phenylalanine-free formula is needed. However, breastmilk has lower levels of phenylalanine than formula milk and, combined with a phenylalanine-free formula, close monitoring and expert support and advice, breastfeeding is possible (Kanufre *et al.*, 2007).

- **Infants may need other food in addition to breastmilk for a limited period if they are:**

  - born weighing less than 1,500g;
  - born less than 32 weeks' gestational age;
  - at risk of hypoglycaemia (preterm, small for gestational age, have suffered a hypoxic episode, are ill infants or infants whose mothers are diabetic, with low blood sugar levels).

This chapter will focus on the issues related to the infant with special needs and some other conditions or situations, such as poor weight gain, hypernatraemia and tongue-tie, that may also pose problems and challenges with breastfeeding.

Learning outcomes

By the end of this chapter you will be able to:

- identify those conditions or situations where breastfeeding may be temporarily challenged;
- provide evidence-based information for mothers to help them maintain lactation when their infant is unwell or if they are separated.

Mapping the UNICEF UK BFI educational outcomes

12 Be able to support mothers who are separated from their babies (e.g. on admission to SCBU, when returning to work) to initiate and/or maintain their lactation and to feed their babies optimally.

14 Identify babies who require a managed approach to feeding and describe appropriate care.

Strategies for care in the neonatal unit

To help neonatal unit staff to provide evidence-based care, UNICEF UK BFI published standards for neonatal care (see Box 1.2 on page 13 and Appendix 5 for further details). This has been a recent addition to the BFI programme and does not yet have a separate accreditation process. To a certain degree, neonatal units come under the best practice standards for maternity units, but the new standards expand on this. A systematic review by Renfrew *et al.* (2009) found that BFI accreditation of the associated maternity unit improved breastfeeding-related outcomes in neonatal units. They also suggest that skilled professional support was more cost-effective than normal staff contact due to the increase in improved neonatal outcomes.

Parents should be provided with evidence-based information about the short- and long-term benefits of breastmilk for infants with special needs, so they can make an informed decision about their choice of infant feeding. However, the principles of supporting breastfeeding for these infants are the same as for healthy term infants:

- early feeding following birth (where clinically appropriate);
- skin-to-skin contact;
- correct position and attachment;
- if the infant is unable to suckle, breastmilk should be expressed and given by an alternative method that will not interfere with future breastfeeding.

Assessing readiness to feed should be based on:

- gestational age;
- physiological status and alertness;
- sucking pattern;
- feeding cues (McGrath and Braescu, 2004).

If the infant is unable to breastfeed or requires alternative methods of infant feeding, this should be discussed with the parents and their decision recorded in the care plan. As with term infants, teats should avoided in case 'nipple–teat confusion' develops (Neifert *et al.*, 1995). A more suitable method of providing nutrition should be used that will not interfere with future feeding at the breast. McInnes and Chambers (2008a) conducted a systematic review of 27 papers to identify interventions to promote breastfeeding or breastmilk feeding for infants admitted to the neonatal unit. The only conclusive interventions that appear to support breastfeeding they could find were skin-to-skin contact, postnatal support and the use of galactagogues. They concluded that there was a lack of research into interventions such as cup feeding and that neonatal unit staff needed to work with individual mothers and infants to determine the most appropriate plan of care. They did, however, highlight that, given the evidence to support the physical and emotional benefits of breastfeeding for the mother–infant dyad, these plans should support mothers to express breastmilk and breastfeed to maximise milk production, increase maternal confidence and promote continued breastfeeding following discharge.

Expressing breastmilk

Most normal healthy infants will demand 8–12 feeds per day within the first 24–48 hours; however, if they are ill, preterm or separated from their mothers they may be unable to do this. Mothers should therefore be encouraged to express breastmilk as soon as possible after birth to stimulate the production of prolactin in order to prime the lactocytes to establish milk production, as well as provide colostrum for the infant. The aim is to establish a milk supply of approximately 750ml/day by day 10. Emphasis should be on frequent expressing and the avoidance of long intervals between expressions.

Chapter 3 explains the technique for hand expression and the use of mechanical breast pumps. Because mothers of ill infants may spend a lot of time in the neonatal unit, it is important to provide a supportive environment, physical and psychological, and to provide facilities that are comfortable for expressing milk, and privacy if preferred. Once discharged from hospital, mothers will express their breastmilk at home and will need clear guidelines

Activity

Can mothers loan breast pumps from your local maternity unit? If not, develop a contact list of agencies that mothers can rent breast pumps from.

about the safe handling, storage and transport of the breastmilk. There should also be a system for the provision of breast pumps for home use while the mother and infant are separated.

'Double pumping' or simultaneous pumping is encouraged as it saves time and increases prolactin levels, and therefore milk production (Renfrew *et al.*, 2009). Both breasts are pumped using a mechanical breast pump for about 10–15 minutes, whereas for single pumping it can take approximately 15 minutes at each breast. Breast massage prior to pumping may increase expressed milk volumes (McInnes and Chambers, 2006). However, McInnes and Chambers (2006) report that some mothers preferred a hand pump to an electrical pump.

Mothers should be instructed to store the required quantity of breastmilk for each feed in a separate sterile container with her name, date, time of expression and unique identifying number. If not used immediately, breastmilk should be stored in a fridge designated for this purpose only. Temperature recordings should be taken daily and should not exceed 2–4°C. Expressed breastmilk should be used within 24 hours or frozen in a freezer at a temperature of –20°C for a maximum of six months (BFN, 2009a). If the mother expresses at home she should follow the same guidelines and transport the breastmilk in an insulated container with ice packs to the neonatal unit.

Activity

What is the local policy for the safe handling, storage and transport of the breastmilk in your neonatal unit?

Skin-to-skin or kangaroo care

Kangaroo care gets its name from the marsupial, the kangaroo, which births its infants at an early gestation and then incubates them by carrying them in a pouch. Kangaroo care was developed in Colombia in response to inadequate resources for ill infants. Instead of having the preterm cared for in an incubator, the infant is cared for next to the skin of the mother or father for a prolonged period of time. The infant is placed skin-to-skin (usually only wearing a nappy and possibly a hat), in an upright position between the mother's breasts or on the fathers chest.

Infants who are separated from their mothers have increased heart rate and blood pressure and higher levels of cortisol. The touch and warmth of skin contact reduces these symptoms and also increases oxytocin levels in infants, which has an analgesic effect. Not only does kangaroo care have a soothing effect on preterm infants by providing comfort, physiological stability and improved sleep, it also encourages bonding, parenting behaviour (Johnston *et al.*, 2008) and increased breastfeeding, by providing easier access to find the breast and attach and allowing the mother to learn feeding cues (McInnes and Chambers, 2008). Even if the infant is unable to suckle, kangaroo care enables the infant to learn to recognise the smell of the mother's skin.

Bergman *et al.* (2004) conducted a randomised controlled trial and found that infants weighing 1,200–2,199g, who had skin-to-skin contact, were more able to maintain their temperature after six hours than those in an incubator (Roller, 2005). A systematic review conducted by Conde-Agudelo and Belizan (2009) supported this, as they also found that kangaroo care reduced severe illness, infection, breastfeeding problems and maternal dissatisfaction with care. However, they also recommend further research in this area of practice. Roller (2005) reports mothers describing kangaroo care as a calming and positive experience for them as well.

The BFI neonatal standards recommend that parents should be informed about the benefits of skin-to-skin contact. It is important that this is carried out in an unhurried environment as soon as the infant's condition allows and should occur as often as possible. Renfrew *et al.* (2009) found that short periods of skin-to-skin contact of up to an hour, at all visits, increased the duration of breastfeeding.

Galactagogues

Some mothers may have difficulty in establishing and maintaining lactation and, in addition to skin-to-skin contact and frequently expressing milk, they may need galactagogues such as domperidone or metoclopramine. Renfrew *et al.* (2009) suggest that this line of treatment is more useful for mothers whose lactation is not meeting the infant's needs rather than for those who have recently given birth. Galactagogues increase prolactin levels by blocking dopamine, which acts as prolactin inhibitor. Unfortunately, they are not licensed to augment lactation and there is a lack of evidence to support dosage. However, the most common dosage is domperidone 10mg or metoclopramine

10mg, taken orally three times a day for up to a week (Jones, 2009c). If this does not work, the dose can be continued or increased (see local guidelines). Once the lactation is established the drug can be withdrawn slowly. Anecdotally, two or three capsules a day of fenugreek may also help improve milk supply, but this should be taken in consultation with a doctor as it can interfere with the action of other medications. Other natural remedies include anise, basil, blessed thistle, caraway, chasteberry and fennel (Jones, 2009c).

Preterm infants

Breastfeeding preterm infants (less than 37 weeks' gestation) can be particularly challenging for mothers and healthcare professionals supporting them, as the infants' needs will vary according to their size, gestation and physiological stability. Preterm infants who are not fed breastmilk are at increased risk of morbidity and mortality. Preterm infants have an immature gastrointestinal tract with increased permeability and susceptibility to infection (Lawrence and Lawrence, 2005). It is therefore extremely important that they are either breastfed or receive breastmilk where possible to provide protection against infection. Breastmilk has high levels of anti-infective properties and prebiotics (good bacteria), which reduce the incidence of necrotising enterocolitis, diarrhoea, respiratory infection and the development of allergies (Henderson et al., 2007). Breastmilk is also more readily digested than formula and has a low renal solute load. Some infants may require prescribed formula fortification of the breastmilk or supplementation if the volumes of expressed breastmilk are insufficient or donor milk is unavailable.

Lactogenesis II is significantly delayed in mothers of extremely premature infants for a number of reasons, such as incomplete mammary growth, and the stress and anxiety that mothers of preterm infants face. Henderson et al. (2008) suggest that lactation can be further reduced in those treated with corticosteroids (betamethasone) in the antenatal period between 28 and 34 weeks' gestation, where birth occurs three to nine days later. This is further compounded if mothers do not express milk more than six times a day. Walker (2010) suggests that poor lactation is indicative of the competition for available insulin by the breasts and the rest of the body. Hartmann and Ramsay (2006) suggest that the shorter length of pregnancy and poor placental function, resulting in a reduction in placental lactogen, may make the situation worse.

These problems are also compounded by the fact that preterm infants:

- have poor or absent suck-swallow-breathe coordination (dependent on gestational age);
- lack 'cheek pads', leading to a weak suck;

- may have nasal prongs, feeding tubes etc., leading to a poor oral experience;
- may have lung disease or other neurological or physical impairments;
- may lack the energy to complete a feed;
- require medically indicated supplementary feeds.

It is therefore imperative that there is a supportive and positive developmental environment that is private, warm and quiet, with reduced light and noise levels, to encourage skin-to-skin contact or kangaroo care. Skin-to-skin or kangaroo care is an important aspect of care for premature infants; not only does it help regulate breathing, heart rate and temperature, it also enhances milk ejection and access to the breast for the infant (Moore *et al.*, 2009). In a randomised controlled trial, Hake-Brooks and Anderson (2008) found that preterm infants, 32–36 weeks, who had unlimited kangaroo care, breastfed for longer than the control group who received traditional nursery care (5.08 months as opposed to 2.05 months).

Interventions may be introduced into neonatal units to encourage preterm infants to suckle. Non-nutritive sucking using dummies may be used in neonatal units to provide comfort, to encourage a sucking technique and to provide a positive oral experience. However, dummies are withdrawn by approximately 32–34 weeks to encourage breastfeeding. Nipple shields may also be used to make it easier for the infant to latch on to the breast. Aloysius and Lozano (2007) conducted a study of 12 mothers, over a one-year period, whose infants were in the neonatal unit and who requested a nipple shield. The reasons for using nipple shields were flat or inverted nipples or the infant being used to a firmer teat. The mothers reported that the shields helped with attachment; however, one discontinued using the shield because she felt it reduced her milk supply and went on to successfully breastfeed. The study concluded that some preterm infants may benefit from the use of nipple shields in the transition period to breastfeeding from tube or bottle feeding and that it may in fact increase milk yield. Further research is required in this area.

Depending on the infant's physical condition and gestation, infants who are unable to suckle at the breast can be given expressed breastmilk by alternative methods such as a nasogastric tube, syringe or cup (see Chapter 8). Although they can suck at the breast from approximately 32 weeks' gestation, the rooting reflex is underdeveloped and they will therefore require additional support with position and attachment (Genna, 2008).

Between 30 and 34 weeks, preterm infants are able to lap milk from a cup, which gives the advantage of providing satisfying oral experience and gastric stimulation. With cup-feeding the infant is able to control the amount and rate of the feed similar to breastfeeding. Therefore, the intake for preterm infants should be monitored over a 24-hour period rather than forcing the calculated amount at each feed. Preterm infants who are cup-fed have higher oxygen saturation levels and are less likely to desaturate during a feed, and also have lower heart rates (Rocha *et al.*, 2002).

By 36 weeks' gestation infants should be able to coordinate the suck-swallow-breathe reflex to feed at the breast (McGrath and Braescu, 2004), but may lack energy to sustain a full feed; in these circumstances the infant may benefit from '*switch nursing*'. Switch nursing or feeding is when the infant is switched from one breast to the other two or three times during each feed as the infant's sucking slows down and swallowing is less frequent. This enables the infant to get the high-calorie milk following a let-down reflex, in order to increase its energy, to enable it to feed for longer and go on to demand feed. There is concern however that the infant does not feed long enough to get the high-fat breastmilk because it may not empty the breast, and switch nursing is therefore only to be used as a temporary measure. Infants who are born small for gestational age are usually very hungry and feed frequently and regularly. Despite this, they may still require breastfeeds to be supplemented to meet the nutritional needs.

Hypoxic infants

Hypoxia can occur at any gestation, either because of an in-utero event or at birth. It is usually caused by placental insufficiency, cord issues or other problems such as meconium aspiration. Asphyxiated infants cannot feed for a minimum of 48 hours and require intravenous fluids until the paediatric team decides milk can be given (Lawrence and Lawrence, 2005). Breastmilk is particularly valuable for infants following a hypoxic event, where the motility of the gastrointestinal tract may have been affected, as it is more easily digested and absorbed while offering anti-infective properties unavailable in formula milk.

As soon as possible after birth the mother should be encouraged to express colostrum, which can be stored for her infant until required; this will also initiate lactation. When possible, skin-to-skin contact should be promoted. When the infant is able to feed at the breast the mother will need skilled support, as these infants often have poor suck-swallow-breathe coordination. Supplementation will be required and a suitable method of administering this should be chosen, avoiding a bottle and teat as these infants are more prone to nipple confusion (Lawrence and Lawrence, 2005). The mother will require help with position and attachment. Lawrence and Lawrence (2005) recommend the 'dancer hold', whereby the mother cups the breast and infant's jaw together in her hand to help form a seal. The use of a sling may be beneficial to support the infant's body at the same time.

Jaundice

Jaundice can be a very complex problem and it is essential that midwives can differentiate between physiological jaundice, breastmilk jaundice and jaundice with a pathological cause. In utero the fetus has high levels of fetal red blood cells, which are no longer required following birth and need to be broken down. The haem component of the red blood cell is converted to biliverdin and bilirubin. Some bilirubin is bound to albumin in the circulation, where it is transported to the liver and conjugated. It is then transported via the bile duct to the intestine to be eliminated in stool. However, some bilirubin remains unconjugated and remains in the system as free-bilirubin, which is reabsorbed. Jaundice is increased in preterm infants due to polycythaemia, following trauma or bruising (forceps or vacuum delivery), infection, metabolic disorders and ineffective feeding.

There are three types of jaundice that the midwife must be aware of and able to diagnose to ensure the correct treatment is initiated: pathological jaundice, physiological jaundice and breastmilk jaundice.

Pathological jaundice presents within 24 hours of birth and is the result of an underlying disease such as haemolytic disease or sepsis. It is essential for these infants to have a paediatric review.

Physiological jaundice is more common and is thought to occur in about 50–60 per cent of infants. It usually presents around the third day following birth, fading gradually over the following ten days. It is also more common in breastfed infants. Physiological jaundice is caused by:

- red blood cell breakdown, leading to increased bilirubin levels and re-absorption;
- reduced albumin levels, reducing the albumin-binding capacity of conjugated bilirubin;
- limited production of glucuronyl transferase to metabolise fat-soluble unconjugated bilirubin to water-soluble conjugated bilirubin;
- enteric reabsorption of unconjugated bilirubin due to delayed clearance of meconium.

Serum bilirubin levels should be taken if the jaundice is significant or the infant appears unwell. If the serum bilirubin in a term infant is above 200μmol/l or 150μmol/l in a preterm infant, or the infant is unwell, the infant should have an urgent medical review and possible treatment with phototheraphy or, in extreme cases, blood exchange transfusion. High serum bilirubin levels can be neurotoxic and lead to kernicterus (a form of brain damage) (Levene *et al.*, 2008).

Breastfeeding has been associated with jaundice; however, Walker (2010) suggests this may be due to poor breastfeeding practices that restrict breastfeeds and encourage maternal–infant separation, with the effect of infrequent breastfeeds, weight loss and delay in meconium evacuation. There appears to be a lack of research related to jaundice and breastfeeding (Renfrew *et al.*, 2005); however, in 2000, Renfrew *et al.* (2000) identified unrestricted feeds, no supplements and rooming-in as effective treatments.

Practice recommendations

- Encourage skin-to-skin contact and rooming in so the mother can pick up infant feeding cues.
- Encourage regular breastfeeds, at no more than three-hourly intervals, to increase bowel motility, clear meconium and reduce the reabsorption of unconjugated bilirubin. Colostrum acts as a laxative, which purges the bowel of bilirubin. If the infant is sleepy it will need to be wakened.
- Observe and assess breastfeeds to ensure adequate milk transfer.
- If the infant has difficulty feeding, weight loss is more than 7 per cent of the birthweight or there are signs of dehydration, the mother should be encouraged to express breastmilk following the feed and give this as a supplement or 'top-up' via a cup or other appropriate alternative feeding method.
- WHO (2003) and NICE (2006a) advise that infants with jaundice should not be routinely supplemented with formula, dextrose and water.

Physiological jaundice can become worse if the infant does not feed frequently. This is further exacerbated by the fact that jaundiced infants tend to be sleepy and reluctant to feed. Mothers need a lot of support with sleepy infants; unlimited skin-to-skin contact for easy access to the breast should be encouraged to facilitate rooting behaviour and prolactin surges for the maintenance of milk production. Regular breastmilk expression should also be encouraged and given to the infant by cup or spoon.

Breastmilk jaundice is normal and can occur as late as ten days after birth and last for several months; its cause is unknown. The infant is asymptomatic and this condition is rarely of concern; however, other causes should be excluded before coming to this diagnosis (Levene *et al.*, 2008).

Hypoglycaemia

Immediately following birth the infant loses its constant glucose supply from its mother and has to maintain its own plasma glucose levels as well as adapt to intermittent nutrition episodes. Blood glucose levels are maintained by insulin and glucagon levels secreted by the islets of Langerhans in the pancreas (see Figure 7.1). In the normal healthy term infant, blood glucose levels will drop to approximately 2.6mmol/l (WHO, 1977) or 2.0mmol/l (NICE, 2008b) (see local protocol) following birth, but gradually rise to approximately 3.6mmol/l after about six hours. Correspondingly, plasma insulin levels decrease following birth, making it more difficult for glucose to be taken up by the cells. In response, glucose serum glucagon levels rise, converting intracellular glycogen stores to glucose (glycogenolysis). The high levels of glucose lead to increased levels of insulin and decreased glucagon levels, but the stores of glycogen will decrease rapidly over the first 24 hours after birth. The newborn also has the ability to mobilise alternative fuels through lipolysis and ketogenesis. This is a normal physiological process and therefore there is no reason to monitor blood glucose levels for the normal healthy term infant within the first two to four hours as it will only encourage unnecessary intervention.

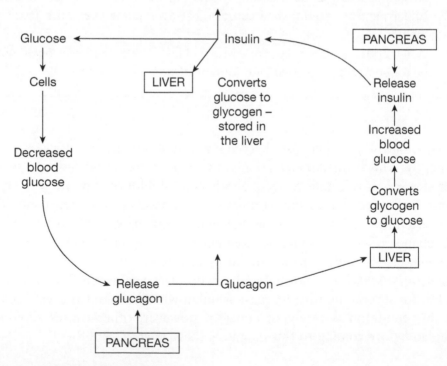

FIGURE 7.1 Glycaemic control

Glucose is essential for brain function, but some infants are at risk of hypoglycaemia (plasma glucose less than 2.6mmol/l) (WHO, 2003; Levene *et al.*, 2008), such as preterm infants; infants who are small or large for gestational age; if there has been birth trauma or hypoxia, infection or hypothermia; and infants of diabetic mothers, and mothers on labetolol prior to giving birth (causing hyperinsulinaemia) (see Chapter 6 for management of the infant of a diabetic mother). These infants must be identified and correctly managed. Signs of hypoglycaemia include lethargy, tachypnoea or apnoea, hypotonia, irritability, unstable temperature, twitching, convulsions or coma. Jitteriness is not an absolute sign of hypoglycaemia as many infants respond like this to handling in the first few days (UNICEF, 2010c).

Practice recommendations (high-risk infant)

The main aim is to avoid hypoglycaemia, first by identifying a 'high-risk' infant and then by providing the appropriate care:

- Skin-to-skin contact whenever possible to encourage breastfeeding and maintain body temperature. Avoiding the infant becoming cold is probably one of the main interventions to prevent hypoglycaemia. Skin-to-skin contact also stabilises the heart and respiratory rate and reduces crying (Moore *et al.*, 2009). All of this avoids the infant using up its glucagon stores too quickly.
- Encourage an early breastfeed within the first hour following birth.
- Breastfeed at least every two to three hours or whenever the infant appears hungry. Breastmilk is thought to improve mobilisation of alternative energy sources.
- The first blood glucose should not be taken before two hours following birth and should be taken prior to the second feed. If a low blood glucose is found before a feed, it should be repeated one hour after the feed (UNICEF, 2010c).
- Regularly monitor vital signs and blood glucose for high-risk infants (see your local protocol). If blood glucose is maintained >2.6mmol/l there is no need for formula milk top-up feeds. However, if the infant is symptomatic, expressed colostrum should be given following a breastfeed via a cup, syringe or nasogastric tube (see Chapter 8). If no breastmilk is available, formula milk can be given at the rate of 8–10ml/kg, preferably by cup (UNICEF, 2010). Some infants may require intravenous infusions.
- Monitor pre-feed blood glucose for 24–48 hours. If plasma glucose levels fall below 2.6mmol/l (see local policy), ensure the infant is given a feed and arrange a paediatric review. If stable on three consecutive occasions after 24 hours, discontinue blood glucose monitoring but continue to observe and provide supplemental feeds until demand feeding is established.

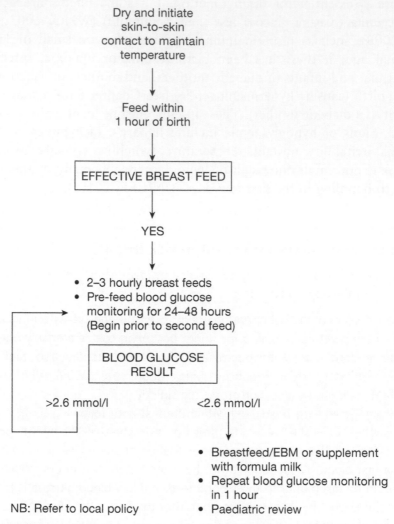

FIGURE 7.2 The management of infants at risk of hypoglycaemia at birth

Postmature infants

Postmature infants have remained in utero as the placental function decreases. They usually have diminished subcutaneous fat, and dry and peeling skin. As well as losing subcutaneous fat, postmature infants have begun to lose glycogen stores and may be hypoglycaemic at birth. Maintaining temperature may be a problem and therefore an early breastfeed and skin-to-skin contact are required to maintain temperature and blood glucose levels (Lawrence and Lawrence, 2005). Due to their lack of glycogen stores, hypoglycaemia may continue to be a problem and therefore blood glucose monitoring may be required (see Figure 7.2). Once established, breastfeeding should not be a problem.

Tongue-tie (ankyloglossia)

Tongue-tie, or ankyloglossia, is when the frenulum (membrane), which holds the tongue in place at the floor of the mouth, is either thicker or shorter than normal and is graded level 1–4, with grade 1 being most severe (Trotter, 2010). When the infant cries the tongue remains fixed to the bottom of the mouth. The tongue has an important role in breastfeeding by positioning the breast in the mouth and creating a vacuum to draw the milk from the breast. Some infants with tongue-tie can breastfeed successfully; however, others may have difficulty attaching to the breast because they cannot open the mouth wide enough to scoop the breast, as the tongue is unable to extend beyond the gum, which in turn affects the tongue's movements when sucking. (This can also be a problem for bottle-fed infants.) This means that milk cannot be effectively removed from the breast and the infant 'nipple-feeds', which will ultimately cause reduced milk supply, nipple damage, pain and an unsatisfied and hungry infant. Blocked ducts, mastitis and abscesses may all be a result of ineffective milk removal. The infant may also go on to have poor weight gain and growth, prolonged jaundice and be introduced to formula milk (Finigan, 2009). Tongue-tie should be noted at the routine examination of the newborn and a plan of care developed to include additional support with position and attachment and, in some cases, surgery.

In cases where breastfeeding is a problem, surgically dividing the tongue-tie is required (Hogan *et al.*, 2005) (see Figure 7.3). Geddes *et al.* (2008) conducted a study to identify whether frenulotomy was an effective treatment for tongue-tie. She used ultrasound imaging before and after surgery to assess the infant's tongue action, milk transfer and milk intake. She found that all measures were improved. However, she recommended that cases be individually assessed prior to treatment.

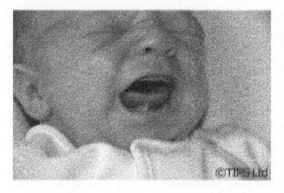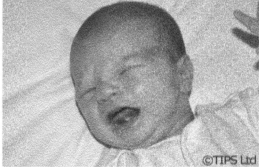

FIGURE 7.3 Tongue-tie (ankyloglossia): (a) before frenulotomy and (b) after frenulotomy
Source: © TIPS Ltd.

Frenulotomy is a quick procedure that, in many cases, does not need a general anaesthetic, but a local anaesthetic is sometimes used. The infant is wrapped up and the tongue-tie divided with sterile blunt-ended scissors (NICE, 2005). The mother is given back the infant immediately following the procedure for a feed. The parents should be advised that there will a few spots of blood only and sometimes a white patch under the tongue that resolves within 48 hours. There is a list of hospitals and contact details where frenulotomy is carried out in the UK on the BFI website (www.babyfriendly.org.uk). Some tongue-ties resolve themselves; however, as the infant gets older it may present problems with weaning and possibly speech.

Weight loss or poor weight gain

Weight loss or failure to gain weight can be an indication of either inadequate milk transfer or underlying illness. If the problem is underlying illness, referral should be made to the paediatrician or GP immediately. A lactation history should be taken to identify problems that may have reduced the milk supply or slowed down the onset of lactogenesis II. The most common cause for poor weight gain or weight loss is ineffective removal of milk from the breast and therefore observation of a breastfeed must be carried out to exclude causes of insufficient milk supply.

Signs of ineffective milk transfer in the infant are:

- weight loss;
- abnormal urine or stool output;
- lethargy and irritability;
- unsettled infant, particularly after prolonged or frequent feeds;
- prolonged or excessive jaundice.

Some of the causes of ineffective milk transfer may be:

- poor position and attachment at the breast;
- lack of stimulation of the breast – scheduled feeding rather than demand, supplementary feeding, use of teats and dummies;
- cracked nipples, mastitis or other common problems;
- maternal issues such as ill health following a traumatic birth or medical problem, Caesarean section, retained placenta, polycystic ovaries, obesity, taking the combined contraceptive pill, substance abuse, previous breast surgery;
- lack of confidence.

Monitoring weight

As a minimum standard NICE (2008c) recommends that normal healthy infants should be weighed naked:

- at birth;
- at the fifth and tenth day as part of the assessment of feeding;
- at two, three, four, eight and ten months (no more than every two weeks).

However, weighing will occur more frequently if the infant is preterm, having feeding problems or has an underlying illness. Iyer *et al.* (2008) found that early weighing with appropriate lactation support resulted in earlier identification of problems, such as neonatal hypernatraemic dehydration, and led to higher breastfeeding rates. Weight loss is calculated as a percentage using the following formula:

$$\frac{\text{weight loss (g)}}{\text{birthweight (g)}} \times 100 = \text{weight loss (\%)}$$

Therefore, if the birthweight is 3800g, the weight loss will be:

$$\frac{200g}{3800g} \times 100 = 5.2\%.$$

The new WHO growth charts include a separate preterm section for infants 32–36 weeks' gestation; a chart for preterm infants born before 32 weeks' gestation; no centile lines between 0–2 weeks; and the fiftieth centile has been de-emphasised (DH, 2009c, p. 5).

Management of weight loss or poor weight gain

Weight loss or poor weight gain of 10 per cent or less

(See local policies as there may be some difference.)

- Take a lactation history and observe a breastfeed and sucking pattern.
- Correct specific problems that have led to weight loss or poor weight gain.
- Encourage prolonged skin-to-skin contact and rooming-in.
- Teach skills of position and attachment, feeding pattern and recognising infant feeding cues.
- Stimulate the breast with regular breastfeeding and/or expressing every two to three hours.

- Supplementary feeds may be required. These should be in the form of expressed breastmilk following a breastfeed where possible.
- Avoid teats and dummies.
- Closely monitor urine and stool output and feeding behaviour.
- Weigh regularly.

Practice recommendations (newborn)

In newborns a normal weight loss is considered to be approximately 5–7 per cent, after which the minimum weight gain should be 20g per day. Excessive weight loss of 7–10 per cent of the birthweight is indicative that the infant is not getting enough milk. If by day 10–14 the infant has not regained its birthweight, the mother should be referred to an experienced infant feeding adviser (Livingstone *et al.*, 2000; Dewey *et al.*, 2005) and should be reweighed every couple of days. If the birthweight has not been regained by the third week, referral to the GP or paediatrician should be made. Clear communication and documentation regarding the plan of care between the healthcare professionals is required as this is often the time when the care of the mother and infant is transferred to the health visitor.

The aim of any intervention is to increase the mother's confidence and motivation to continue breastfeeding, to address and correct the identified problem and prevent further complications.

Weight loss of 10–12 per cent

- As above.
- Refer to paediatrician or GP as appropriate.
- Encourage mother to express milk after every feed at the breast and then cup feed. Formula milk may be required if insufficient breastmilk is available.
- Weigh in 24 hours.

Weight loss greater than 12 per cent

- As above.
- Refer to neonatal unit and paediatric staff.
- To be seen by an experienced infant feeding adviser.

If weight loss is above 15 per cent, an emergency paediatric review is required. A full biochemical profile for electrolytes and renal function will be performed as well as a renal ultrasound. If the infant is able to breastfeed this should continue; however, intravenous fluids will also be required. The mother should be reviewed by a skilled breastfeeding adviser and encouraged to express breastmilk every two to three hours.

Activity

Ensure you are familiar with your local policy for weighing infants and the referral process should it be required. What are the differences in the policy for normal healthy term infants and those in the neonatal unit?

Practice recommendations (older infant)

In the first four months of life an infant will gain approximately 125–200g per week. This will slow down to 50–150g by four to six months and 25–75g by six to twelve months. This will vary between infants, but similar methods of ensuring the newborn is thriving can be applied to the older child:

- the infant is active and alert;
- at least six wet nappies a day;
- frequent stools;
- good signs of position and attachment at the breast.

Poor weight gain can be attributed to underlying illness; however, it is more commonly due to poor breastfeeding technique or problems with lactation. Management will include a full lactation history, observation of position and attachment, monitoring of urine and stool output, observation of feeding behaviour, and skilled help and support. Skin-to-skin contact and co-bathing should be advised at any age to encourage feeding behaviour. The mother may also need to increase the number of times she breastfeeds and to express following a feed to increase her milk supply (see Chapter 3).

Hypernatraemic dehydration

All infants are expected to lose weight within the first few days of life, which is thought to be due to fluid loss. A normal weight loss is currently considered to be up to 7 per cent of the birthweight. Extreme weight loss is, however, associated with hypernatraemic dehydration – increased blood sodium levels – and is usually caused by insufficient feeding (Livingstone *et al.*, 2000; Dewey *et al.*, 2005).

All healthcare professionals must be aware of the signs of hypernatraemia:

- weight loss;
- abnormal pattern of wet and dirty nappies;
- lethargy or irritability;
- fever;
- jaundice.

It must be noted that newborn infants with hypernatraemic dehydration do not always display the classical signs of dehydration, for example increased skin turgor, sunken fontanelle, sunken eyes, dry mucous membranes, increased capillary refill time and cool/blue peripheries. These may all be absent but the infant may still be dehydrated. It is therefore essential to teach mothers what the normal pattern of feeding is and what they can expect. Infants over 48 hours old usually feed approximately eight times in 24 hours (hypernatraemia is rare in infants <48 hours old).

Livingstone *et al.* (2000) give the risk factors for hypernatraemic dehydration as:

Infant
- abnormalities of the mouth;
- preterm infants;
- use of teats or pacifiers;
- birth trauma;
- medical problems;
- separation from mother;
- sleepy baby.

Mother
- breast problems such as cracked nipples, hypoplasia;
- complicated birth;
- delayed lactogenesis II;
- postpartum haemorrhage;
- infrequent breast stimulation.

Livingstone *et al.* (2000) recommend that, if infant weight loss is greater than 7 per cent and continues to fall within the first week of life, or the birthweight has not been regained by the tenth day, referral should be made to a skilled infant feeding adviser for the early detection of insufficient milk transfer and the prevention of hypernatraemic dehydration.

Vitamin D supplementation

There has been great debate in recent years regarding whether or not breastfed infants require vitamin supplementation, in particular vitamin D. Vitamin D is predominantly produced photochemically in the skin by exposure to sunlight and is available in a few foods (e.g. fish oils, liver, dairy products). Due to concerns about vitamin D deficiency, some countries fortify foods such as cereals, bread and margarine.

Vitamin D regulates calcium phosphate, which is essential for the development of healthy bones. It is associated with protection against prostate and colon cancer, psoriasis and a number of autoimmune disorders, and a reduction in the incidence of type 1 diabetes. Deficiency, however, is associated with increased susceptibility to tuberculosis, cardiovascular disease, some cancers and osteomalacia. In infants a deficiency results in rickets and continues to be a problem in some high-risk groups (SACN, 2007b). People with darker skin pigmentation such as Black or Asian ethnic minority groups, and those with lifestyle and cultural practices that reduce the amount of time their skin is exposed to sunlight, are at greater risk of vitamin D deficiency (Ladhani *et al.*, 2004; NICE, 2008a).

In 2003, NICE guidelines stated that there was not enough evidence to support routine supplementation of vitamin D for pregnant and lactating women. However, the Scientific Advisory Committee on Nutrition have debated this recommending that this group of women should consider taking a vitamin D supplement of 10 micrograms per day (SACN, 2007b). Based on this advice, NICE updated their antenatal guidelines in 2008 and stated that:

> All women should be informed at the booking appointment about the importance for their own and their infant's health of maintaining adequate vitamin D stores during pregnancy and whilst breastfeeding. In order to achieve this, women may choose to take 10 micrograms of vitamin D per day, as found in the Healthy Start multivitamin supplement. Particular care should be taken to enquire as to whether women at greatest risk are following advice to take this daily supplement.

> (2008a, p. 92)

Those who do not qualify for healthy start vitamins can buy them from a pharmacy.

Practice recommendations

As breastmilk contains low levels of vitamin D it is important to ensure that breastfed infants are not susceptible to vitamin D deficiency. A few simple measures can be recommended:

- Safe exposure to sunlight – approximately 15 minutes three times a week from April to September for people with fair skin and slightly more for those with darker pigmentation (avoid excessive exposure to sunlight to minimise the risk of skin cancer) for mother and infant. In colder climates during winter there is not enough sunlight to maintain vitamin D levels.
- For pregnant and breastfeeding women 10 micrograms daily vitamin D supplementation is recommended. Those in high-risk groups may be prescribed 20 micrograms per day.
- All children over the age of six months until their fourth birthday should be given vitamin supplementation.
- Breastfed infants over one month whose mothers are at high risk of vitamin D deficiency may be prescribed vitamin drops (such as abidec or dalivit).

For further information see www.healthystart.nhs.uk.

Discharge planning

Support with breastfeeding must continue following discharge from the neonatal unit. An individualised care plan should be developed prior to discharge and communicated to the healthcare team that will be providing future care and support; this may be the midwife or health visitor. Any equipment such as breast pumps, storage bottles and sterilising equipment should be in situ before the infant goes home, and the mother should have been shown how to work and maintain the pump as well as safely express and store breastmilk. Follow-up appointments should be made to assess feeding and to ensure the infant is thriving. The mother should also be informed about other mechanisms of support, such as help-lines, support groups, peer supporters and specialist infant feeding advisers (see Chapter 10).

Concluding comments

There are many situations where breastfeeding can be challenging, but this is particularly the case when the infant has special needs or requirements. It is clear from the evidence that breastmilk offers protection from further illness and healthcare professionals must offer a coordinated approach to care both in the hospital environment and on discharge home.

Scenarios

What would you recommend in the following situations?

1   Amy is three days old and has been prescribed phototherapy for jaundice. Her mother, Carol, informs you that Amy is not feeding well and a friend has advised her to give formula milk as well as breastfeed to clear the jaundice.

2   Ingrid has come to you today. Her baby, Gemma, is 10 weeks old. Gemma was 3.5kg born at 40 weeks' gestation, on the fiftieth centile. Now Gemma's weight is 4.5kg, which is on the ninth centile. Ingrid says feeding is erratic and Gemma has to be 'topped up' with formula milk, as the feeds are sometimes 'frantic' and she keeps coming off the breast.

Further reading

- Hake-Brooks, S. and Anderson, G. (2008) 'Kangaroo care and breastfeeding of mother–preterm infant dyads 0–18 months: a randomised controlled trial', *Neonatal Network*, 27: 151–9.
- Iyer, N., Srinivasan, R., Evans, K. *et al.* (2008) 'Impact of early weighing policy on neonatal hypernatraemic dehydration and breastfeeding', *Archives of Childhood Disease*, 93(4): 297–9.
- Livingstone, V., Willis, C., Abdel-Wareth, L. *et al.* (2000) 'Neonatal hypernatraemic dehydration', *Canadian Medical Association Journal*, 162(5): 647–52.
- McInnes, R. and Chambers, J. (2008) 'Infants admitted to neonatal units – interventions to improve breastfeeding outcomes: a systematic review 1990–2007', *Maternal and Child Health*, 4: 235–63.
- NICE (2005) *Division of Ankyloglossia (Tongue-tie) for Breastfeeding*, Ipg149, London: NICE.
- SACN (2007) Update on Vitamin D: Position statement by the Scientific Advisory Committee on Nutrition 2007, London: The Stationery Office.

Chapter 8 Alternative methods of infant feeding when breastfeeding is not possible

- Learning outcomes
- Supplementary and complementary feeding
- Alternatives to breastfeeding
- Donor milk
- Formula feeding
- Sterilisation, preparation and reconstitution of formula milk
- Concluding comments
- Reflective questions
- Resources

It must be acknowledged that, in some circumstances, breastfeeding is not possible for mothers or infants. This chapter will cover a range of alternative feeding methods and the use of donor milk when the mother's own breastmilk is not available. Safe artificial feeding will also be described and instruction on sterilising feeding equipment included.

Learning outcomes

By the end of this chapter you will be able to:

- identify alternative methods of infant feeding when feeding at the breast is not possible, including the use of expressed breastmilk, donor breastmilk and formula milk;
- discuss the risks and benefits of alternative methods of feeding;
- demonstrate how to feed an infant safely with these alternative methods;
- demonstrate how to prepare formula milk safely and sterilise feeding equipment.

Mapping the UNICEF UK BFI educational outcomes

13 Be able to demonstrate a knowledge of alternative methods of infant feeding and care which may be used where breastfeeding is not possible and which will enhance the likelihood of a later transition to breastfeeding.

The best way for infants to receive breastmilk is to suckle at the breast. However, sometimes breastfeeding is not possible due to a variety of reasons such as illness, prematurity or separation from the mother. It is therefore essential that healthcare professionals not only have a sound knowledge of the available alternative methods of feeding, but also know how to assess the appropriateness for the gestational age and clinical condition of the infant.

Nipple–teat confusion is a major concern for healthcare professionals (Renfrew *et al.*, 2000) and can be defined as the interference of artificial nipples, such as teats and dummies/pacifiers, with the successful initiation of

Table 8.1 Suggested feeding devices suitable for gestational age and feeding behaviour

Gestational age	Feeding behaviour	Suggested feeding device for supplement
<30–32 weeks	Uncoordinated suck-swallow-breathe reflex	Intravenous gastric tube
30–32 weeks	Can 'lap' milk	Drops of milk; cup feed
32 weeks	Begins to suckle at the breast but requires supplementation	Cup feed; supplementer
34–36 weeks	Increasing amounts from breast	Cup feed

breastfeeding. It is this idea that forms the basis of Step 9 of the UNICEF *Ten Steps*: '*Give no artificial teats or dummies to breastfeeding infants*'. It is clear that there is a difference in the mechanism of sucking an artificial teat and the breast; however, there is limited evidence to support the avoidance of teats or dummies in healthy term infants and much of the research available is based on premature infants or infants with other compounding factors (Hargreaves and Harris, 2009) rather than healthy term infants.

STEP 9: Give no artificial teats or dummies to breastfeeding infants.

In a randomised controlled trial of 700 breastfed infants, Howard *et al.* (2003) found that dummies had a detrimental effect on breastfeeding, as did supplemental feeds. However, they also identified some benefits for infants born by Caesarean section or those requiring regular supplementation. Cup feeding was also found to increase the length of postnatal stay in hospital in this study. The BFI acknowledged the findings of this study but continue to recommend that Step 9 remains, suggesting an 'open mind' until further research is undertaken. As there is no way of determining which infants will develop nipple–teat confusion, it is appropriate to avoid artificial teats where possible and use other devices until the infant is able to feed from the breast, for example by nasogastric tube, cup, spoon or supplementer.

Supplementary and complementary feeding

Supplementary and complementary feeding are terms that are often used interchangeably, but they mean very different things. In some literature, 'supplementary' means giving a feed in place of a breastfeed, whereas 'complementary' means topping up a breastfeed with expressed breastmilk, formula or even water. The following BFI definitions are used in this book:

- *Supplementary feeding*: Feeds given to a infant under six months old to supplement the intake of breastmilk, where this is insufficient.
- *Complementary feeding*: The introduction of foods and drinks after six months of age. These foods are in addition to an adequate intake of breastmilk.

The reasons for giving supplementary feeds include medically indicated reasons, lack of evidence-based practice or parental choice. The *Infant Feeding Survey 2005* (Bolling *et al.*, 2007) identified that, in the UK, 35 per cent of mothers gave their infant formula milk at birth. This is of concern, as only 24 per cent did not initiate breastfeeding at birth. Therefore, approximately 11 per cent or just over 1 in 10 breastfeeding mothers gave formula on the first day. They also found that 45 per cent of mothers were exclusively breastfeeding at one month, but this figure reduced to 21 per cent at six weeks, and to less than 1 per cent at six months. By four weeks, 32 per cent of mothers had given additional drinks to their infants and this rose to 84 per cent by six months. Breastfed infants were less likely than formula-fed infants to have additional drinks. The most common reasons for giving additional feeds were because the infant was thirsty, constipation, colic/wind/indigestion and to settle the infant.

> **STEP 6/POINT 5**: Give newborn infants no food or drink other than breastmilk, unless medically indicated.

A study by Tender *et al.* (2009) found that 78 per cent of infants received supplementation while in hospital and the reasons for only 13 per cent of these were based on policy. They reported that the reasons for supplementation were mothers' perception that their infants were not getting enough milk by breastfeeding alone or that the milk was 'not in'. Professionals reported that they were allowing the mother to rest or that the mother was on medication. Alarmingly, 20 per cent of the mothers in this study did not know why their infant had been given a supplement. They also reported that those mothers who did not receive antenatal education were 4.7 times more likely to receive supplementation.

> **STEP 3/POINT 4**: Inform all pregnant women about the benefits and management of breastfeeding.

If supplementation is considered necessary it must be preceded by careful assessment, taking a lactation history and observing a breastfeed. Breastmilk should always be used as the preferred option to formula milk where available.

To guide healthcare professionals, the WHO and UNICEF (2009) published the following guidelines for acceptable medical reasons for giving breastmilk substitutes:

- **Infants with the following conditions cannot have breastmilk and require specialised formula milk**:
    - galactasaemia (need galactose-free formula);
    - maple syrup urine disease (need formula free of leucine, isoleucine and valine);
    - phenylketonuria (breastfeeding is possible but they also need phenyl-alanine-free formula and close expert monitoring). (See Chapter 6 for further details.)

- **Infants may need other food in addition to breastmilk for a limited period if they are**:
    - born weighing less than 1,500g;
    - born less than 32 weeks' gestational age;
    - at risk of hypoglycaemia (preterm, small for gestational age, have suffered a hypoxic episode, are ill infants or infants whose mothers are diabetic, with low blood sugar levels). (See Chapter 7 for further details.)

If the mother is HIV positive, breastfeeding should be avoided if suitable alternatives are available (see Chapter 6). Some other conditions require breast-feeding to cease temporarily, but it can resume if or when there is a change in status, for example: severe illness such as sepsis; herpes simplex lesions on the breast; taking medications such as sedatives, anti-epileptic drugs and other drugs that could cause drowsiness; and radioactive iodine or chemotherapy (see Chapter 6).

Other issues that could indicate supplementation are geographic separation, delayed lactogenesis II, severe nipple pain, breast anomalies or previous breast surgery, infant dehydration, weight loss of more than 7–10 per cent of the birthweight and meconium still present at five days (Walker, 2010).

To ensure lactation is maintained and improved in these situations, mothers should be encouraged to have skin-to-skin contact, attempt to breastfeed where possible and express breastmilk after the attempted breast-feed to encourage prolactin production and avoid a build-up of the FIL (see Chapter 2), which will reduce the milk supply and trigger apoptosis.

Alternatives to breastfeeding

Nasogastric tube feeding

Nasogastric tube feeding is used to provide breast or formula milk for premature or ill infants where the infant cannot maintain its nutritional needs via the breast or bottle alone; or due to a lack of ability to suckle adequately. The nasogastric tube delivers the milk straight into the stomach and therefore the infant does not have the oral stimulus of the feed. It is preferable if a bolus feed is administered during kangaroo care or when the infant is at the breast, even if the infant cannot suck, so that it associates the feed with the breast.

Procedure for inserting the tube and delivering the milk

- Measure the tube from the tip of the xiphisternum to the tragus of the ear (tough fold of cartilage at the entrance to the ear) and to the nostrils.
- The infant should be relaxed.
- Insert the tube slowly to avoid vagal stimulation and resulting bradycardia.
- Check for gastric aspirate using pH indicator paper to ensure the tube is in the stomach not the lungs. Gastric contents should be pH 5.5 or less. Above 6 could indicate the tube is in the intestines; pH above 7 could indicate the tube is in the lungs and must be removed.

Once it has been confirmed that the tube is in the correct position, feeding can commence. An oral syringe should be used to administer the feed. The milk should be delivered using gravity, not pushed down the tube with a plunger.

Cup feeding

From approximately 30 weeks' gestation, infants have the ability to lap milk from a cup. The advantages of cup feeding for preterm infants above other methods such as a nasogastric tube are that it provides oral and gastric stimulation. The infant experiences taste and also demonstrates tongue movement. With cup feeding the infant is able to control the amount and rate of the feed similarly to breastfeeding, therefore the intake for preterm infants should be monitored over a 24-hour period rather than forcing the calculated amount at each feed. It is also important to note that, compared to bottle feeding, preterm infants who are cup-fed have higher oxygen saturation levels, and are less likely to desaturate during a feed, and they also have lower heart rates (Rocha *et al.*, 2002). However, cup feeding is not appropriate for all infants; it is unsuitable for infants who have a poor gag reflex or are lethargic, as they are likely to aspirate.

Flint *et al.* (2007) conducted a review of four studies that compared cup and bottle feeding. They found that, although three of the studies demonstrated that infants who were cup-fed rather than bottle-fed were more likely to be exclusively breastfeeding at discharge, there was no difference at two and six months. They also found the length of postnatal stay in hospital was increased in those who were cup-fed; however, this could have been because it was policy not to allow infants home if they were still cup feeding.

Procedure for cup feeding

- Wrap the infant and support the infant in an upright position.
- Half fill the cup with breastmilk or formula.
- Bring the brim of the cup to the outer corners of the infant's upper lip, resting on the lower lip.
- Tip the cup to ensure the milk is touching the infant's lips so that it can lap or sip the milk. Do not pour the milk into the mouth.
- Allow the infant to regulate the pace but avoid the feeding session taking over 30 minutes.
- Keep the cup in position while the infant rests.
- Wind the infant at regular intervals.

Syringe

Small doses of approximately 0.5ml via a 1ml syringe may be suitable for the infant who can swallow but not suck; any amounts greater than this should be administered via a cup to avoid aspiration.

Procedure for syringe feeding

- Wrap the infant and support the infant in an upright position.
- Deliver very small amounts of milk into the cheek area of the mouth.
- Allow time for the infant to swallow and take a breath in between each dose.

Breastfeeding supplementer

The supplementer is a fine tube that, when attached to the breast, is used to supplement feeding during a breastfeed. As the infant takes the breast into its mouth it also takes the tube. As the flow of milk at the breast is stronger than the tube, the infant first empties the breast and then receives the prescribed supplement. The benefits of this device are that it enables the infant to suckle at the breast and obtain breastmilk on demand, providing a positive feeding experience for mother and infant while stimulating lactogenesis.

The supplementer facilitates delivery of nutrition for the infant while stimulating the breast to produce milk and is therefore suitable for mothers with insufficient milk supply, those who have had prior breast surgery, to help induce lactation or relactation, and for mothers with premature infants or infants with disorders, illness or neurological impairment that cause a weak suck.

Procedure for using the breastfeeding supplementer

- Use a fine tube such as a nasogastric tube and a cup or bag for the milk (expressed breastmilk where possible).
- Place one end of the tube along the nipple so that the infant suckles the breast and tube at the same time.
- Place the other end of the tube in the cup of milk or attach to the bag.
- Control the milk flow by raising the cup to increase the flow and lowering it to decrease the flow.
- Thoroughly clean the equipment between each use by boiling or sterilising or, if in hospital, use single-use equipment.

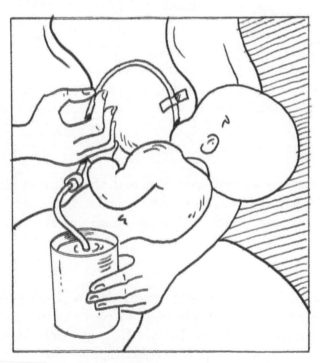

FIGURE 8.1 A breastfeeding supplementer

Finger feeding

Finger feeding is where a feeding tube is attached to the finger and inserted in the infant's mouth. It is a useful method for mothers who experience breast refusal or whose infant is sleepy, has latching problems or is premature with suckling difficulties. It is most commonly used to prepare and encourage the infant to feed at the breast.

Procedure for finger feeding

- Use a suitable container to hold the milk and attach the tube securely.
- Place the tube so that it is placed on the soft part of the index (or other) finger.
- The end of the tube should go no further than the end of the finger. Taping it to the finger may help it maintain position.
- Wrap the infant and support the infant in an upright position.
- Using the finger with the tube attached, gently touch the infant's lips until it opens its mouth. The infant should begin to suckle.
- The soft part of the finger should be flat and face upwards towards the roof of the mouth.
- If feeding is very slow, the container may be raised above the infant's head.

Haberman feeder

A Haberman feeder is a special bottle developed for infants with impaired sucking ability (for example, cleft lip and palate). It is designed to mimic breastfeeding as opposed to sucking on a traditional artificial teat and bottle.

Dropper/pipette

These devices may be used to drop milk on to the breast to encourage the infant to suckle or lick at the breast. This is useful for reluctant feeders and premature infants who are unable to suck, and to encourage the let-down reflex.

Donor milk

Donor milk banking was established to collect, screen, pasteurise and distribute donated breastmilk for infants whose mothers are unable to breastfeed or supply their own breastmilk. In 2010, NICE developed donor breastmilk guidelines aimed at professionals who either support mothers who use donor milk, work in a donor milk bank or intend to set up a donor milk bank.

At the time this document was published there were only 17 donor breastmilk banks in the UK who supplied breastmilk predominantly for infants requiring neonatal care (see Appendix 6). The United Kingdom Association for Milk Banking (UKAMB) is a registered charity that supports donor milk banking and is a useful resource for parents and professionals (see www.ukamb.org).

Potential donors have to go through a rigorous screening interview and serological testing at enrolment. Donors are given information on the processes and how the breastmilk will be used, and are informed that it will not be returned to them. Informed consent is gained before any breastmilk is provided.

During the screening interview the donor is asked if she smokes; drinks more than two units of alcohol twice a week; uses or has ever used recreational drugs; has ever tested positive for HIV, hepatitis B or C, human T-lymphotrophic virus or syphilis, or is at increased risk of Creutzfeldt-Jacob disease. If she answers yes to any of these questions she is not allowed to donate her breastmilk. If she answers no to the questions she undergoes serological screening and another interview. Donors require ongoing training, support and assessment of health and serological status. They are advised to contact the milk bank if they develop pyrexia, take medication or develop any breast infection, including mastitis.

NICE *Clinical Guideline 93* (2010) (http://guidance.nice.org.uk/CG93) provides further information.

Training for donors includes:

- the importance of hand washing and good technique;
- personal hygiene;
- expressing and collecting breastmilk;
- cleaning and using breast pumps;
- storing breastmilk (including labelling and documentation);
- transporting the breastmilk.

Donors are encouraged to express milk by hand and collect the expressed milk rather than 'drip' milk (milk that drips from one breast while the infant is feeding at the other).

The NICE guideline (2010) provides strict criteria for the storage, collection, transport and processing of donor milk. The donor milk is pasteurised at 62.5°C for 30 minutes and can be stored for no longer than six months. Good documentation of all the processes is kept for 30 years after the expiry date. Donor breastmilk is only supplied to hospitals that agree to comply with the tracking process.

Donor milk usually comes from mothers who have given birth at term. Therefore, the milk content tends to be variable in relation to fat, energy and protein content and alone may not meet the nutritional requirements of preterm or low birthweight infants. However, donor breastmilk does have the advantage of providing the immunoprotective factors and growth factors that may prevent necrotising enterocolitis. Quigley *et al.* (2007) conducted a systematic review and found that, although there were greater short-term growth rates in those preterm infants fed with preterm formula, it was associated with an increased incidence of necrotising enterocolitis.

Administering donor milk in the neonatal unit

All donor breastmilk (or mothers' own expressed milk) should be checked by two members of staff beside the infant, immediately prior to administration. The infant's name and identifying number should be checked against the milk and the infant. The staff should also ensure that consent has been gained from the parents. The consent form, alongside the donor milk record sheet, should be kept with the infant's case record and a copy sent to the donor milk bank for tracking purposes.

Activity

Does your local neonatal unit use donor breastmilk? Read the local policy and guidelines as there may be slight variation in procedure.

Formula feeding

Although breastmilk is the gold standard for infant nutrition, some mothers are unable to, or choose not to, breastfeed or express breastmilk for their infants. The only alternative to breastmilk suitable for infants under one year is formula milk (SACN, 2008a). It is therefore essential that healthcare professionals support these mothers and have knowledge about formula milks. At times, the message from UNICEF UK BFI has been misconstrued and some healthcare professionals falsely believe that the BFI does not allow them to advise and support women who choose to bottle feed. In fact, this is not the case and the BFI website (www.babyfriendly.org.uk) supplies advice sheets for parents who choose to bottle feed and for healthcare professionals to enable them to provide consistent and evidence-based information. Also, as part of the accreditation process, they have included the requirement that all mothers who choose not to breastfeed are able to correctly prepare a bottle of infant formula before discharge (UNICEF, 2010e). Cairney and Alder (2001) conducted a study involving 365 postpartum mothers in which 50 per cent of the mothers reported that they had not been given information about safe techniques for bottle feeding. In addition, approximately 65 per cent of breastfeeding mothers who introduced bottle feeding at a later date did not remember getting any information either.

Formula milks are designed to be similar to breastmilk. However, because of the nature of breastmilk (see Chapter 2), formula milk cannot replicate it fully. Most formula milks are developed from cow's milk; however, soya milk is also available to parents. The content of formula milk is regulated by statute in *The Infant Formula and Follow-on Formula Regulation 2007, European Community Regulations 2006/141/EC.* Despite this, there are some variations in the permitted content between formula brands and these can cause intolerance in some infants. If this is the case, mothers can change the brand, usually under the advice of the midwife or health visitor.

Types of formula milk

Preterm milk

These products are designed to provide nutrients suitable for preterm infants and are enriched with proteins and minerals.

First milks

These are for newborns and are based on the whey of cow's milk at a ratio of 60:40 whey:casein which is similar to breastmilk. Whey-dominant formula is more easily digested than casein-dominant formulas. This should be suitable for most infants until they are six months old and can be continued while the infant is being introduced to solid food until the age of one year, when it can start drinking full-fat cow's milk.

Second milks

The main difference from first milks is that second milks are casein dominant, the ratio being 20:80 whey:casein. Second milks are marketed for 'hungry infants' and manufacturers state that they *can* be given to newborns but the high casein ratio, which is supposed to make the infant feel full and settle more easily, makes them more difficult to digest and they are therefore not usually recommended for newborns by healthcare professionals. Health Scotland (2010) recommends continuing whey-based formula milk until the age of 12 months.

Follow-on milks

These milks are marketed as suitable for infants over six months of age and should never be used in younger infants. They contain more iron, sugars and minerals than first milks. There is no evidence to suggest any benefits for infants moving to follow-on formula at six months and therefore it is not recommended (SACN, 2007a; Health Scotland, 2010; UNICEF, 2010d).

Goodnight milks

These milks are marketed for infants between the ages of six months and three years and contain follow-on milk with rice flour, whole-grain oatmeal and corn starch. They can be given via a bottle or feeding cup. Again, on behalf of the Department of Health, the SACN (2008a, p. 3) could find no evidence to support manufacturers' claims that they 'settle the infant for the night' or are 'gentler on the infant's tummy'. The SACN (2008, pp. 3–4) identified some other concerns about these milks:

- They may replace the night breastfeed, therefore undermining continued breastfeeding.
- Going to bed immediately after such a feed could result in prolonged tooth exposure to the food and lead to dental caries. (The manufacturers do recommend brushing the teeth before bed; however, this seems to contradict the notion of 'settling' the infant.)
- Some parents may use these formula feeds to settle the infant at other times of the day and this may interfere with weaning. The SACN suggests that they are not a suitable alternative to meals.
- The preparation of goodnight milks is different from those of other formula milks and may cause confusion for parents.

Soya milk

This is made from soya beans and is not advised as an alternative milk for infants; it should only be used under the advice of the GP or health visitor. Despite common perception, infants who are allergic to cow's milk may also be allergic to soya milk (FSA, 2010b) and it cannot be recommended for the prevention of allergies (Osborn and Sinn, 2006). Soya milk contains high levels of phytoestrogen, which may pose long-term reproductive problems. It may also cause problems for infants with hypothyroidism and stimulate allergies. Soya milk contains more sugars from non-milk sources and can therefore lead to dental caries. Martyn (2003) suggests that infants of parents who are vegans are most at risk, as they may assume that the infant will get the same benefits as adults.

Other formula milks

Goat's milk formula is not suitable for infants. Hypoallergenic formulas for infants with a proven cow's milk intolerance or at risk of allergies should be used under medical or dietetic consultation.

Full fat cow's milk

This should not be given to infants under one year of age.

Constituents of formula milk

- *Long-chain fatty acids* are found in breastmilk and are thought to improve brain and eye development. Formula manufacturers introduced them into their milk and use this to market their products. However, Simmer *et al.* (2008) found no evidence of benefit when added to formula.
- Infant formula companies have introduced *prebiotics* into their milk in an attempt to encourage the growth of 'good bacteria', bifidobacteria and

TABLE 8.2 Comparison of breast and formula milk (adapted from RCM, 2009)

Nutrient	Breastmilk	Formula milk
Fat	Omega DHA, AA	No DHA
	Cholesterol	No cholesterol
	Lipase	No lipase
	Adjusts to infants needs, reducing as infant gets older	Does not adjust
Protein	Increase in whey (easy to digest)	Increase in curds (harder to digest)
	Lactoferrin (binds iron)	No lactoferrin
	Lysosomes	No lysosomes
	IgA	No IgA
Carbohydrate	Lactose (important for brain development)	Deficient in lactose
	Rich in oligosaccharides	Deficient in oligosaccharides
Other	Taste varies	Taste never varies

lactobacilli in the digestive tract, or the good bacteria itself in the form of *probiotics*. However, Osborn and Sinn (2007) could not find sufficient evidence to support the use of prebiotics and probiotics in formula milk.

- *Nucleotides* make up the units of DNA and RNA and are thought to enhance gastrointestinal and immunological effects.
- *Vitamins A and D* are added to formula milk, including special preterm products, and therefore exclusively formula-fed infants under six months of age do not require these supplements. Those over the age of six months and up to the age of two years will require vitamin A, D and C supplements. However, groups at high risk of vitamin D deficiency should still take the supplements (see Chapter 7) (UNICEF, 2010d).
- Formula milk has 5–6 times more *iron* than breastmilk, but because it is 'free iron' it is less bio-available or readily absorbed and increases the risk of infection.

Advice for parents

The preparation and reconstitution of formula milk, as well as the timings and quantities, can be of great concern to parents, especially if their infant does not adhere to the guidelines on the packet. The BFI (2010b) recommends that all infants, whether breast or formula-fed, should be fed on demand. In the first few days infants may only take a small amount of formula, but by the end of the first week they will require approximately 150–200ml/kg/day until they are six months old. Parents need advice that they should not overfeed their infant in the hope that it will go longer between feeds, as the infant is likely to vomit and also put on too much weight. Teaching parents the signs to look for when the infant is hungry is helpful.

Signs of hunger

- Moving the head from side to side, with the tongue protruding.
- Sucking fingers.

Parents should not wait until the infant cries as it will become frustrated and not feed as well. It is also important to reinforce to the parents that formula-fed infants' sleep patterns may change, particularly during growth spurts, but that this does not mean that the milk needs to be changed or that weaning should commence; the infant may just require a greater number of feeds for a few days.

Many parents worry about the amount of milk the infant drinks and particularly if it is getting enough. They should be taught the signs of adequate feeding to look for:

- at least six wet (soaked) nappies a day; clear or pale urine;
- sticky meconium for the first few days of life followed by pale yellow/yellow-brown stools at least once a day.

The infant's weight should be plotted on the new growth chart at regular intervals and discussed with the parents (DH, 2009c).

Many parents who formula feed are concerned about constipation and resort to old wives' tales as remedies. Renfrew *et al.* (2003) reported that reconstitution errors are the most common cause of constipation, by putting too much powder in the bottle compared to the volume of water. If this is not the cause, changing the brand of milk may be a solution, as the hardness of the stools is related to unsaturated fatty acids in the stools. This should be discussed with the health visitor. There is no evidence to support giving additional water to improve constipation.

Equipment

Many bottles and teats are designed to replicate the breast; however, this is impossible given the unique nature of the anatomy of individuals' breasts. However, parents do seek advice on these products. The BFI advice sheet (2010d) recommends that milk should drop out of the teat of an upturned bottle at one drop/second. If the flow is too fast it will spill out of the infant's mouth and, if too slow, the infant may become frustrated.

Sterilisation, preparation and reconstitution of formula milk

Powdered formula milk is not sterile (ready-to-use cartons are) and can become contaminated by pathogens such as *Enterobacter sakazakii* and *Salmonella*. In the past 40 years there have been between 50 and 60 known cases of infection from powdered formula milk; preterm and low birthweight infants are most at risk (FSA, 2010a). The Food Standards Agency (FSA) recommends that healthcare professionals should re-emphasise the importance of good hygiene practices in the preparation and storage of feeds to reduce the risk of illness.

Sterilising feeding equipment

- Wash hands with soap and water.
- Wash feeding equipment in hot soapy water.
- Bottle and teat brushes should be used to clean inside teats and bottles to remove all traces of the formula milk.
- Rinse equipment under a running tap.
- Sterilise equipment using preferred method and following manufacturer's guidelines.
- Leave the bottle until time to make up a feed or fully assemble the bottle with the teat inside and lid on to prevent contamination.
- Wash hands and clean preparation surface where formula milk will be reconstituted.

There are different ways to sterilise infant feeding equipment (DH, 2007a), such as cold-water sterilising and steam sterilising. Manufacturers' guidelines should be followed. Renfrew *et al.* (2008) conducted a systematic review to assess the clinical and cost-effectiveness of different methods of cleaning and sterilising infant feeding equipment at home. They concluded that there was a lack of evidence to suggest which method is most effective. However, they did emphasise the importance of hand washing before handling the equipment.

Preparation of a formula feed

The DH (2007a) recommends that only one bottle of formula should be made up immediately before a feed, as storage of reconstituted powdered milk may enhance the likelihood of becoming contaminated by pathogens such as *E. sakazakii*, thus increasing the risk of illness.

- Clean the preparation area and wash hands with soap and water.
- Boil fresh tap water in a kettle and allow it to cool to no less than 70°C (less than 30 minutes), because at this temperature it will kill most bacteria.
- Pour the required amount of water into the sterilised bottle.
- Add the exact amount of formula to the water as per manufacturers' guidelines. The wrong amount could cause electrolyte imbalance; too much may cause constipation and dehydration and too little could cause malnutrition.
- Reassemble the bottle and shake well to ensure the powder has reconstituted.
- Quickly cool under a running cold tap or in a container of cold water.

- The temperature should be lukewarm; test a few drops on the inside of the wrist.
- Discard any formula that has not been used within two hours.

However, if parents are unable to follow best practice for any reason (for example, leaving the house, taking bottles to nursery), it is important that they are given advice to prepare and store feeds as safely as possible. The FSA (2010a) recommends reducing the storage time where possible, but suggests the following options:

- use prepacked cartons of liquid formula (sterile); or
- put the boiled water into a vacuum flask and use it to make up the feed fresh at the time it is required.

If this is not possible parents should be advised as follows:

- If more than one feed is required, always prepare them in separate bottles as stated above, not in one container.
- Store the bottles in the back of a fridge, not the door, at a temperature below 5°C. (*E. sakazakii* and *Salmonella* can grow in reconstituted formula if stored above this temperature.)
- The fridge temperature will need close monitoring if the fridge is opened frequently.
- The less time the feed is stored, the less risk of contamination by pathogens; this time should never exceed 24 hours in the fridge.

When reheating the bottle if stored in the fridge:

- Only remove from the fridge when required.
- Place in a container of warm water for no longer than 15 minutes; never reheat in a microwave as this causes hot spots.
- Shake the bottle to ensure it has reheated evenly and test a few drops on the inside of the wrist to make sure it is lukewarm.

If the parents need to transport a prepared bottle feed, it should have been in the fridge for at least one to two hours at less than 5°C and immediately placed in a cool bag with ice packs. It must be used within four hours. If transported in less than four hours, it should be placed in a fridge at less than 5°C and used within 24 hours. However, this should be avoided where possible and is only advised in exceptional circumstances, as it increases the risk of contamination by pathogens and resulting ill health.

The *Infant Feeding Survey 2005* (Bolling *et al.*, 2006) reported that just under half of mothers who had prepared formula feeds in the last seven days had not followed the recommendations for preparing formula milk and admitted they did not always use boiled water that had been cooled for less than 30 minutes. Nor did they always add the powder to the water and instead did it the other way around. Approximately one third of mothers admitted to not following the recommendations for preparation or storage of formula milk when away from home.

Advice for bottle feeding an infant

- Hold the infant close.
- Keep the infant in an upright position with its head supported.
- Brush the teat over the lips and wait until there is a wide gape and the tongue is in the base of the mouth before putting the teat in the mouth.
- Position the bottle horizontally and tilt it so that the infant can get the milk from the teat and not air, which will cause wind.
- Bubbles will be seen in the bottle if the infant is feeding well.
- Allow the infant to have short breaks; it may need to wind occasionally.
- Never leave the infant unattended with a bottle.

Concluding comments

Although breastfeeding should be the norm for human infants, some infants or mothers are unable to, or choose not to, breastfeed. Healthcare professionals have a duty of care to ensure they can support these mothers to use alternative methods to meet the nutritional needs of the infant. For some, this is a temporary situation due to illness or separation. Therefore, careful consideration must be given to the method of providing nutrition so that it is not detrimental to later breastfeeding success. Unfortunately, many parents who choose to formula feed over breastfeeding complain that they are not taught the technique of bottle feeding by healthcare professionals (Cairney and Alder, 2001). This can have detrimental consequences for the health of the infant and it is therefore imperative that midwives ensure that mothers are able to feed their infants confidently before being discharged from the hospital (UNICEF, 2010e).

Reflective questions

- How do you decide what alternative method of feeding can be used for infants who are temporarily unable to breastfeed?
- What education do you provide for mothers, before discharge from hospital, who choose to formula feed their infants?
- How do you keep up to date on changes in formula milk and feeding equipment?

Resources

- *Donor Breastmilk Bank: The Operation of Donor Milk Banks Services*
  www.guidelines.nice.org.uk
- NHS bottle-feeding guidance
  www.nhs.uk/Planners/birthtofive/Pages/bottle-feeding.aspx
- A full list of all the infant formulas available in the UK in 2003 can be found at:
  www.sacn.gov.uk/pdfs/smcn_03_06.pdf
- UNICEF UK BFI guidance for formula feeding
  www.babyfriendly.org.uk/items/resource_detail.asp?item=627
- United Kingdom Association of Milk Banks (UKAMB)
  www.ukamb.org

Chapter 9 **Introducing solid foods**

- Learning outcomes
- Introducing solid food
- Advice on food types for parents
- Concluding comments
- Scenario
- Further reading

Mothers need evidence-based advice and support to ensure that the timing of introducing solid food is appropriate and safe and does not incur any health problems. The WHO (2002) recommends exclusive breastfeeding for the first six months of life and to continue alongside other foods for two years (see Chapter 1). This chapter aims to be a practical guide to introducing infants to solid food.

Learning outcomes

By the end of this chapter you will be able to:

* discuss the appropriate time to introduce solid foods;
* describe the signs of developmental readiness for the introduction of solid foods;
* identify the appropriate foods to introduce during weaning.

Mapping the UNICEF UK BFI educational outcomes

10 Understand the importance of timely introduction of complementary foods and of continuing breastfeeding during the weaning period, into the second year of life and beyond.

Introducing solid food

Introducing solid food before six months is not recommended because there is insufficient developmental readiness to cope with foods other than breast or formula milk. The aspects of developmental readiness relevant to introducing solid foods are:

* development of the infant's immune system;
* maturity of the gastrointestinal tract and kidneys;
* oral development and ability to chew;
* hand-to-mouth coordination.

The WHO (2002) and the DH (2008) recommend the gradual introduction of solid foods at six months for both breastfed infants and those who are formula-fed. In addition, mothers need to be taught to recognise the signs to look out for that suggests their infants are ready to be weaned:

* they can maintain an upright sitting position on their own;
* they mimic the family eating;
* they can grab food and put it in their mouths;
* they can swallow the food.

This should be followed by accurate advice and support on how to do this safely. Weaning should be a gradual process, while breastfeeding continues on

> **Key fact**
>
> The World Health Organization (WHO, 2002) recommends that infants should be exclusively breastfed until the age of six months because:
>
> - breastmilk provides all the nutrients an infant requires for the first six months of life;
> - breastfeeding reduces the incidence of gastrointestinal, respiratory and ear infection;
> - breastfed infants are less likely to develop type I and II diabetes or become obese;
> - the longer the mother breastfeeds, the less likely she is to develop pre-menopausal breast cancer and osteoporosis, and the quicker she will return to her pre-pregnancy weight;
> - menstruation and the return of fertility are delayed with exclusive breast-feeding.

demand. As the infant adjusts to the changed regime and new tastes and textures, another meal can be introduced. By the age of one year, the infant should be having three meals a day and eating a varied diet, supplemented with either breast or formula milk. Mothers should be encouraged to continue breastfeeding as long as the child requires (DH, 2008).

By eight to nine months the infant should be taking three meals a day, be used to a range of soft and mashed foods and be introduced to soft finger foods. By 10–12 months the infant should be eating chopped food rather than mashed, as well as firmer finger foods such as fruit or bread sticks. From 12 months on the infant should be fitting in with family meals (DH, 2009b). See www.nhs.uk/start4life/pages/taste-for-life.aspx or www.healthscotland.com/resources/publications for further detail.

Baby-led weaning

Rapley (2006) suggests that introducing infants to a variety of foods can be achieved by a common sense approach she termed 'baby-led weaning'. Her theory was based on her observations during a small study in 2005 of five breastfed infants who were introduced to solids at four months of age (in line with recommendations at the time) and is based on the infants' development over the first year. At approximately six months, the digestive tract and immune system are ready for the introduction of other foods and the infant

Practice recommendations (gradual weaning)

- Start slowly with simple, natural foods such as mashed vegetables, fruit or cereal mixed with milk (breast or formula) or fist-sized soft fruit or vegetables.
- Once the infant is used to these tastes and textures, other healthy food can be introduced such as meat, fish and pasta.
- Allow food to cool, testing the temperature before giving to the infant.
- Let the infant feed itself as it is normal for infants to play with food to discover new textures and tastes; mothers must be prepared for the mess.
- Provide a variety of tastes and textures.
- Do not hurry the process of weaning; each infant will progress at an individual pace.
- Do not leave infant alone while eating because of the risk of choking.
- Continue to observe nappies for urine output to avoid dehydration.

is able to sit up, grab food and put it in the mouth and chew. She acknowledged parents' concerns about choking, but reassured them that this should not be a worry if the following safety guidelines are adhered to:

- The infant should be sitting upright.
- Only the infant should put food in its mouth.
- Do not leave infants alone with food.
- Remove stones from fruit.
- Do not give the infant nuts.

Rapley (2006) suggested that almost all food types can be introduced to the infant after six months of age alongside breastfeeding or formula feeding (see 'Advice on food tips for parents' below). She recommended initially giving foods that can be easily cut up into hand-held sizes, long enough for some to protrude from the infant's fist, so the infant can hold it. She advises parents not to worry about the amount of food taken in the first few months, as breast or formula milk will provide adequate nutrition; early introduction to solid food should be fun and a learning experience. The following guidelines are adapted from Rapley's (2008) leaflet, *Baby-led Weaning*:

- Sit the infant upright facing a table.
- Offer food rather than feeding it to the infant.

- Start with food that is easy to pick up (hand-held size).
- Involve the infant at family meal times and, if suitable, offer the same food.
- Choose meal times when the infant is not tired.
- Continue breast or formula milk feeds but not necessarily at meal times.
- Offer water with meals.
- Do not hurry the process.
- Allow the infant to control the amount it wants to eat.

Advice on food types for parents

The aim of weaning is to introduce infants to the variety of foods that the family eats. However, the *Infant Feeding Survey 2005* (Bolling *et al.*, 2007) reported that those mothers who introduced solid food before six months of age were more likely to use manufactured foods, whereas those who weaned after eight months were more likely to introduce home-prepared foods. Mothers should be given the following advice for preparing a healthy diet:

- Avoid foods high in salt, such as cheese, bacon, sausages and processed food not specifically prepared for infants, such as cereals and sauces, because the infant's renal system cannot process them.
- Avoid adding sugar to foods and drinks because it can cause tooth decay and encourages a 'sweet tooth'.
- Honey should be avoided in food for infants less than one year old because of the risk of bacteria that could cause infant botulism. It also has the same issues as sugar (see above).
- Breastfed infants do not require additional drinks; however, formula-fed infants usually do and should be offered cooled boiled tap water or boiled bottled water that states that it is safe for infants. Caution must be taken with bottled water as not all mineral water is suitable for infants.
- Fruit juice diluted (1:10) with cooled boiled water may be given to infants over six months of age with a meal. However, because it contains sugar, which may cause tooth decay, it should be avoided at other times.
- Other drinks that contain sugars should be avoided to prevent tooth decay, particularly if given in a bottle, such as fizzy drinks, squash or flavoured milk. These additional drinks may also inhibit appetite and cause loose stools.
- Cow's, goat's and sheep's milk should not be given as a drink to infants under one year as they do not contain the required nutrients.
- Tea and coffee are not suitable drinks as they inhibit iron absorption.

If the mother decides to begin weaning before the recommended six months, the DH (2008) and Health Scotland (2010) recommend that certain foods, which may increase the risk of allergies, should be avoided, such as:

- bread, rusks and some cereals (gluten);
- eggs;
- fish and shellfish;
- nuts and seeds;
- soft and unpasteurised cheeses.

Concluding comments

The decision of when to introduce solid food is a complex process for mothers and can be positively or negatively influenced by partners, family, friends and healthcare professionals, as well socio-cultural traditions, as discussed in Chapter 1. Therefore, it is essential that healthcare professionals have the knowledge and skills to advise mothers confidently on how to recognise when their infant is ready for solid food, how to go about introducing it, and what types of food to include in a healthy balanced diet.

Scenario

Leasa is a first-time mum. She is worried about her four-month-old baby, Molly. She is gaining adequate weight but has started waking up twice during the night for a breastfeed when she had previously only woken once. Leasa's friends and relatives have advised her to introduce some solids to help her settle through the night.

What would you say to Leasa to reassure her, and what advice would you give her about her decision to introduce solids at this stage?

Further reading

- DOH (2009) Taste for Life, www.nhs.uk/start4life.
- DOH (2010) Breastfeeding and Introducing Solid Foods: Consumer insights summary, London: DOH. See also www.dh.gov.uk.
- Gill Rapley's Baby-led Feeding website www.rapleyweaning.com

Chapter 10 **Ongoing support for breastfeeding mothers**

- Learning outcomes
- Breastfeeding support
- Returning to work
- Sexual activity
- Family planning: lactational amenorrhoea method
- Breastfeeding during pregnancy: tandem nursing
- Relactation or induced lactation
- Concluding comments
- Reflective questions
- Resources

Breastfeeding mothers need ongoing support from professionals, their peers and society in general to continue breastfeeding for as long they would like to. Although many of the issues that influence duration of breastfeeding have been discussed throughout this book, this chapter will focus on particular issues such as accessing different types of support, returning to work and assisting mothers with relactation or induced lactation, family planning and breastfeeding during pregnancy.

Learning outcomes

By the end of this chapter you will be able to:

- discuss the need for ongoing professional, social and peer support;
- advise mothers about both the legal and practical aspects of returning to work;
- assist mothers who have ceased breastfeeding to relactate or to induce lactation in those who wish to breastfeed;
- provide advice about family planning, sexual activity and breastfeeding during pregnancy.

Mapping the UNICEF UK BFI educational outcomes

8 Be equipped to provide parents with accurate, evidence-based information about activities which may have an impact on breastfeeding.

9 Understand the importance of exclusive breastfeeding for the first six months of life and possess the knowledge and skills to enable mothers to achieve this.

11 Understand the importance of community support for breastfeeding and demonstrate an awareness of the role of community-based support networks, both in supporting women to breastfeed and as a resource for health professionals.

12 Be able to support mothers who are separated from their babies (e.g. on admission to SCBU, when returning to work) to initiate and/or maintain their lactation and to feed their babies optimally.

It is clear throughout this book that the evidence supports the fact that breastmilk is the best form of nutrition for human infants and has positive health benefits for both mother and infant, and the longer the infant is breastfed the greater the benefits are. The *Infant Feeding Survey 2005* (Bolling *et al.*, 2007) demonstrated that the breastfeeding initiation rate for the UK was 78 per cent in England, 70 per cent in Scotland, 67 per cent in Wales and 63 per cent in Northern Ireland. However, this was followed by a rapid decline over the first few weeks. They found that 48 per cent of all mothers were breastfeeding at six weeks postpartum, and 25 per cent at six months. However, only 48 per cent of all mothers were exclusively breastfeeding at one week, and only 25 per cent of these were still exclusively breastfeeding at six weeks, and this figure dropped to less than 1 per cent at six months. These figures are alarming and are a long way from meeting the WHO (2002) and DH (2003b) recommendations for exclusive breastfeeding for six months and to continue for two years and beyond. Bolling *et al.* also reported:

> Nine in ten mothers who gave up breastfeeding within six months would have preferred to breastfeed for longer, this level declining as breastfeeding duration increased. Although even among those who breastfeed for at least six months, 40 per cent would have liked to continue.
>
> (2007, p. x)

Bolling *et al.* (2007) identified young mothers, those from lower socio-economic groups and those with lower levels of education to be least likely to commence breastfeeding and those who do breastfeed do so for a shorter duration and are more likely to wean before six months of age. Evidence suggests that a lack of access to appropriate information is a major contributing factor and that the reasons women gave were embarrassment, lack of support and conflicting advice from healthcare professionals. As these women are the least likely to breastfeed, the cycle of deprivation continues and the SACN (2008b) recommends that these groups be 'targeted' for healthcare policies and interventions, and that health professionals and peer supporters should be trained to meet the needs of this vulnerable group.

McInnes and Chambers highlighted that, in general, mothers reported that 'a lack of breastfeeding knowledge acted as a barrier to their receiving and accepting postnatal support' (2008b, p. 423). This is supported by O'Brien *et al.* (2009), who identified that the strategies mothers used to successfully breastfeed included increasing breastfeeding knowledge, goal-setting and challenging unhelpful beliefs. However, as demonstrated throughout this book, the factors that influence the initiation and duration of breastfeeding come from international, national and regional levels as well as from the individual (Dyson *et al.*, 2006). Table 10.1 summarises these issues.

Breastfeeding support

Professional support

McInnes and Chambers (2008b) conducted a review of qualitative literature to produce a synthesis of mothers' and healthcare professionals' experiences and perceptions of breastfeeding support. They concluded that mothers did not receive the support they wanted from healthcare professionals and that healthcare professionals were not the main source of postnatal support; instead, social support was considered to be of greater value. Both mothers and professionals reported that poor staffing levels in postnatal wards resulted in conflicting advice and in a lack of information and support. They suggest that conflicting advice and poor techniques may be a result of a lack of education and training and recommend practical skills training, updates, mentoring and assessment for staff, as well as the need to include interpersonal and communication skills. Building a therapeutic relationship is important when providing support for breastfeeding, as mothers are more receptive if they feel comfortable asking questions and do not feel judged. Practical and consistent advice and information, encouragement and emotional support are crucial elements in developing this relationship, as is continuity of care or carers where possible.

Social support

Mothers are more likely to breastfeed if they have a supportive social network. According to McInnes and Chambers (2008b, p. 422), support with breastfeeding can be split into three categories:

- *practical*   housework, caring for other children;
- *information*   knowledge of breastfeeding;
- *emotional*   empathy, approval, praise, feeling nurtured.

Social support depends on the societal norms for infant feeding and the knowledge, views and beliefs of family and friends. A supportive family network is considered essential for some mothers to overcome challenges they may face. Mothers also value support from those they perceive as 'role models' or who have had experience of breastfeeding, often their own mothers.

Although McInnes and Chambers (2008b) suggest that mothers value support from those with experience of breastfeeding, fathers also play an important role. Where this was positive towards breastfeeding, fathers were able to provide practical, physical and emotional support in the decision to breastfeed as well as to support continuation (Sheriff *et al.*, 2009). However, some men lack knowledge about breastfeeding and believe it will interfere with their relationship, particularly with regard to sex (Hewitt, 2008). In western culture, breasts are often portrayed as sexual objects and are often discussed as the 'man's property' (Dickens, 2008).

It is clear that family and friends also need to be educated about the benefits of breastfeeding and the risks of formula feeding, so that they can provide adequate support for breastfeeding mothers. Many hospitals and community areas have developed innovative ways of doing this, from inviting fathers and prospective grandparents to breastfeeding classes, to developing posters to

TABLE 10.1 Examples of factors (often interrelated) that influence infant feeding at international, national, regional and individual levels

International and national factors	National and regional factors	Individual factors – amenable to medium- to long-term change at the macro socio-economic level	Individual factors influencing decision to breastfeed – amenable to change in the short term at the micro socio-economic level	Individual factors influencing a woman's decision to stop breastfeeding before she wishes – amenable to change in the short term at the micro level
Globalisation of formula feeding in developed countries promulgated by commercial interests	Lack of importance/ understanding of breast-feeding in the organisation of health services; embedded practices or routines that interfere with successful breastfeeding	Maternal age – younger mothers are less likely to breastfeed	Attitudes of partner, mother and peer group	Mother's or health professionals' or family's perception of 'insufficient milk'
Cultural shift to regimented feeding patterns and growth monitoring based on formula feeding regimes	Lack of appropriate education and training for health and related professionals	Maternal education – breastfeeding rates are lowest among those who left school at 16 or less	Social support provided by woman's partner, family and friends	Painful breasts and nipples; baby would not suck or 'rejected the breast'
Increase in work opportunities for women without supportive childcare/ feeding facilities	Lack of integration across sectors – acute, community, social services, voluntary	Socio-economic status of mother (and partner) – breastfeeding rates become lower for lower socio-economic groups	Loss of collective knowledge and experience of breastfeeding in the community, resulting in a lack of confidence in breastfeeding	Breastfeeding takes too long, or is tiring

TABLE 10.1 *continued*

International and national factors	National and regional factors	Individual factors – amenable to medium- to long-term change at the macro socio-economic level	Individual factors influencing decision to breastfeed – amenable to change in the short term at the micro socio-economic level	Individual factors influencing a woman's decision to stop breastfeeding before she wishes – amenable to change in the short term at the micro level
Media portrayal of bottle feeding as the norm and as safe	Lack of supportive environments outside the home and in the workplace	Marital status Ethnicity – cultural tendency for white women to choose not to breastfeed	Whether mothers were breastfed themselves as babies	Mother or baby is ill Difficult to judge how much baby has drunk
Increased media portrayal of women's breasts as symbols of sexuality	Lack of breastfeeding education in schools	Biomedical factors (parity, method of delivery, infant health)	Embarrassment about, difficulty in, or perceived unacceptability of, breast-feeding in public, both in and outside the home, especially for younger mothers	Baby can't be fed by others
Lack of full implementation of WHO Code of Marketing of Breast-milk Substitutes		Return to work before the baby is four months old	Difficulty of involving others, especially partner, in feeding Perceived inconvenience of breastfeeding and anxiety about total dependence of the baby on the mother	

Source: Dyson *et al.* (2006, p. 17).

inform fathers of the benefits (Hewitt, 2008), to campaigns such as the 'Be a Star' campaign, aimed at increasing the number of breastfeeding young mothers by showcasing them as confident women. 'Be a Star' produces posters and radio advertisements and has a website with useful information and tips aimed at all the family (www.beastar.org.uk).

However, if the social network is unsupportive, breastfeeding can be easily undermined and mothers may feel pressurised into stopping breastfeeding or develop a lack of confidence in their ability. Some will seek out other forms of social support, such as peer support groups, and will join voluntary organisations. This was highlighted as particularly important when information was not forthcoming from healthcare professionals or they were unable to help solve problems (McInnes and Chambers, 2008b).

Peer support

Peer support programmes were originally set up in areas of deprivation with poor breastfeeding rates. They either provide support on a one-to-one basis or to groups of women. Mothers appear to value face-to-face contact rather than telephone support (McInnes and Chambers, 2008b). The aim is to improve breastfeeding rates in local communities by putting mothers in touch with other mothers with breastfeeding experience, who can provide support, encouragement and practical advice. The intention is that a peer supporter will have similar demographic characteristics and understanding of the cultural expectations within the local area. Peer supporters receive training but are encouraged to refer complex problems to healthcare professionals. However, this training appears to be different throughout the UK. Dykes (2005) found that the role of listener and confidence builder was more prominent in England and the mechanics of breastfeeding more prominent in Scotland. There was also limited emphasis on building relationships and developing communication skills in most areas. Britten *et al.* (2006) also found a difference in the perceived roles of peer supporters, from friend and role model to breastfeeding expert, which changes the relationship from an equal partnership to one where the supporter has the power, suggesting that roles need to be more clearly defined to avoid confusion with healthcare professionals' roles.

A number of studies have been carried out since the introduction of peer supporters, demonstrating varying success of programmes (Muirhead *et al.*, 2006); however, Renfrew *et al.* (2005) suggest that peer support is effective in increasing the duration of breastfeeding for those who intended to breast-feed, if it is offered soon after birth. Furthermore, Briton *et al.* (2007) claim that peer support combined with professional support is most effective. NICE (2006b, 2008b) recommend that commissioners and managers of maternity units should introduce breastfeeding peer support groups and, in 2010, NICE published a new commissioning and benchmark tool for peer support programmes for women who breastfeed (www.nice.org). The Health Promotion Agency in Northern Ireland (2004) also recommends that peer support be used as a multifaceted approach and that volunteers and healthcare professionals must be proactive in making contact with mothers. It is evident from the literature, however, that further research is required about peer support groups to evaluate their cost-effectiveness and value to mothers.

Activity

- Find out what peer support programmes are available in your area and what the mechanism for referral is. How do women know about them?
- How do you educate family and friends about breastfeeding to support breastfeeding mothers?

Other support organisations

Midwives and other healthcare professionals should be familiar with the national and local breastfeeding support organisations. Some examples of such organisations are:

- **Association of Breastfeeding Mothers (ABM)**
  ABM was established in 1980 by mothers to give other mothers support and accurate information about breastfeeding.

- **La Leche League (www.laleche.org.uk)**
  The La Leche League was formed in 1956 by seven mothers who wanted to support breastfeeding friends. Today they have branches in over 60 countries and their aim remains the same: to offer accurate mother-to-mother breastfeeding support. The organisation is predominantly run by volunteers who lead local groups. As well as providing training for breastfeeding supporters, La Leche also publishes valuable information for mothers and healthcare professionals; many will be familiar with *The Breastfeeding Answer Book*, which is a valuable resource in many healthcare settings.

- **National Childbirth Trust (NCT) (www.nct.org.uk)**
  The National Childbirth Trust is a UK organisation and was formed in 1956. Volunteers provide support for breastfeeding mothers through training and education for parents, counsellors and health professionals.

- **Breastfeeding Network (BFN) (www.breastfeedingnetwork.org.uk)**
  The Breastfeeding Network is a recognised Scottish charity. Its aim is to promote breastfeeding, disseminate accurate, evidence-based information to parents and health professionals, and set standards for breastfeeding support.

- **UNICEF Baby Friendly Initiative (BFI) (www.babyfriendly.org.uk)**
  The UNICEF Baby Friendly Initiative predominantly promotes best practice for breastfeeding mothers within healthcare and higher education settings and offers assessment and accreditation to acknowledge that these institutions achieve high standards. It also provides information for parents; however, it is unable to offer this on an individual basis.

- **Baby Café Charitable Trust (www.thebabycafe.co.uk)**
  Baby Café 'drop-ins' were developed in 2005 and are part of the Baby Café Charitable Trust network run by paid facilitators (voluntary or healthcare professionals). They usually open once a week in a variety of venues and promote open access for all pregnant and breastfeeding mothers.

- **Little Angels (www.littleangels.org.uk)**
  Little Angels was founded in 2004 by mothers who identified a need for local breastfeeding support. It is now a Community Interest Company funded by service-level agreements, contracts and grants. Little Angels provides peer support from the local community.

Activity

There are numerous voluntary organisations throughout the UK to support breastfeeding mothers.

- Do you know the groups in your area of practice?
- Prepare a list of local groups that you can give to mothers in your care.

Returning to work

Many mothers want to continue breastfeeding after they return to work but often perceive this as a barrier to continuing breastfeeding. The benefits of continuing breastfeeding in line with the WHO recommendations (exclusive breastfeeding for six months and to continue for up to two years) for mothers and infants are well known, but there are also benefits for employers. Health Scotland (2009, p. 12) states that these are:

- reduced parental absence as breastfed infants are less likely to be ill compared to formula-fed infants;
- lower recruitment and training costs;
- recruitment incentives;
- increased staff morale.

Legislation

Employers are legally bound to facilitate continued breastfeeding outside normal break times. It is best if this is planned in advance and employers are notified in writing before the mother returns to work so that preparations can be made. The following legislation protects breastfeeding mothers.

Management of Health and Safety at Work Regulations 1999 (2000 Northern Ireland) and Employment Rights Act 2002

The employer has a duty to carry out a risk assessment to assess whether working conditions are a risk to the health of the breastfeeding mother or infant. Some employers may not appreciate the dangers of not breastfeeding and therefore the mother may provide them with some literature.

If a risk is identified, it is the employer's responsibility to reduce the risk (see www.hse.gov.uk/pubns/indg373hp.pdf). This may include temporarily adjusting the mother's working conditions and/or hours of work; or if that is not possible, offering her suitable alternative work (at the same rate of pay) if available; or suspending her from work on paid leave for as long as necessary to protect her health and safety and that of her child (HSE, 2010). If working hours need to be changed, for example to avoid night shifts, this request can be supported by a medical certificate from the GP. If no alternative work schedule can be found, the employee can be suspended on full pay.

Workplace (Health, Safety and Welfare) Regulations 1992

The Workplace Regulations require employers to provide suitable rest facilities for workers who are pregnant or breastfeeding. Ideally, these should be private, have hand-washing facilities and include facilities for the storage of breastmilk.

EU Council Directive 92/85/EEC

This directive is for those working in the public sector. If the employee's work causes problems with breastfeeding, the employer must change the working conditions/hours for as long as she is breastfeeding.

Sex Discrimination Act 1975 (1976 Northern Ireland)

If a woman is required to work particular hours without justification or has unfavourable conditions for breastfeeding, it can be considered as indirect discrimination.

Maternity Leave and Parental Rights 2003

Statutory maternity leave is for 52 weeks. This is 26 weeks of ordinary maternity leave (when a mother is entitled to all her contractual rights such as annual leave) and 26 of extra maternity leave (partially paid).

Both parents are allowed up to 13 weeks' unpaid parental leave per child until its fifth birthday, if they have worked one year by the date they wish to take it. This can follow maternity leave but requires 21 days' notice.

Practicalities of returning to work

Mothers may choose different options for providing their infants with breastmilk while they are at work:

- Express breastmilk and leave it for a carer to give the infant. This may mean expressing milk during working hours, which will also maintain lactation and prevent the breasts becoming overfull.
- Use childcare facilities near the workplace so that they can either breastfeed during the day or immediately before or after work.
- Negotiate shorter or flexible work hours.

The Health and Safety Executive (HSE, 2009) has produced a useful leaflet for new and expectant mothers who work, which can be found at www.hse. gov.uk/pubns/indg373.pdf.

Expressing milk at work

Mothers should not be expected to express milk in the toilet or other unsuitable environment. A clean, warm and comfortable room should be made available with hand-washing facilities and somewhere to store equipment. If a fridge is not available, breastmilk should be stored in a cool bag. Depending on facilities, a mother may use a hand or electric pump or hand express. See Chapter 3 for further details about expressing and storing breastmilk.

Sexual activity

It is suggested that breastfeeding mothers are more keen to resume sexual activity than non-breastfeeding mothers following birth (Lawrence and Lawrence, 2005), but this is not the case for all. Some mothers report milk ejection during sexual activity and increased vaginal dryness. If the milk ejection is a problem for the couple, the mother can wear a bra with breast pads. For vaginal dryness she should be assured that this is due to inhibited hormones during lactation. Vaginal dryness can lead to discomfort during intercourse and a lubricant can be used as a temporary solution.

Family planning: lactational amenorrhoea method

Lactational amenorrhoea method (LAM) is a natural method of family planning. During breastfeeding, prolactin inhibits the release of gonadtrophin-releasing hormone and levels of oestrogen and progesterone are reduced, inhibiting ovulation. It is thought that LAM is 98 per cent effective in the first six months postpartum (Lawrence and Lawrence, 2005), however it is reliant on:

- exclusive and regular breastfeeding;
- the infant being less than six months old;
- there having been no menstrual bleeding after 56 days postpartum.

If these factors do not apply, the mother should not rely on breastfeeding alone as a method of contraception and will require advice on appropriate alternative contraceptives. The progesterone-only contraceptive pill may be used when breastfeeding but the combined oestrogen-progesterone pill must be avoided because it will reduce milk supply.

Breastfeeding during pregnancy: tandem nursing

Many mothers will, however, become pregnant while breastfeeding and may express concerns that they will have to wean the infant from the breast despite wanting to continue. Many mothers are misinformed and told they will have to stop breastfeeding; however, there is no danger to the fetus and breastfeeding can continue in most cases. Advice should be sought if the mother has had a previous miscarriage or preterm birth or experiences bleeding. There is no evidence to suggest that the oxytocin released during breastfeeding will cause the uterus to contract, as oxytocin receptors in the uterus are inhibited until near term. Mothers will need support and advice regarding taking adequate rest and appropriate diet, given the additional demands on them both physically and psychologically.

Some mothers complain of tender nipples during pregnancy and therefore attention to position and attachment is required. Also, during the second and third trimester, the milk changes to colostrum (Lawrence and Lawrence, 2005) to prepare for the new infant. The milk volume decreases and it changes in taste and smell, which may encourage the breastfeeding infant to stop breastfeeding independently. Abrupt weaning initiated by the mother should be avoided, but if the mother intends to wean once the new infant is born this should be a gradual and planned process. The La Leche League recommends the 'don't offer, don't refuse' approach (2006). However, many infants will be happy to continue to breastfeed like this and it must be remembered that many of the benefits of breastfeeding are dose-related.

Once the new infant is born it should be fed first, because an adequate supply of colostrum is essential for newborns and the older infant is getting nutrition from other sources at this point.

Relactation or induced lactation

Relactation or induced lactation is the stimulation of the breast to lactate to breastfeed an infant where pregnancy has been absent, or to restimulate lactation following cessation of breastfeeding (Worgan, 2002). Some mothers may have a reduced milk supply or have discontinued breastfeeding for a variety of reasons and regret the decision. It is important that healthcare professionals are aware that this situation is reversible and develop the skills to enable the mothers to lactate and commence or recommence breastfeeding.

The aim is to trigger the release of prolactin and oxytocin to commence milk production; however, for some mothers not all the prolactin receptors will have been primed initially and therefore full production may not be possible. Inducing lactation requires great commitment and therefore the mother should be very motivated and made aware that it may take a few weeks to establish adequate milk production. Skilled help and support from professionals is required to teach the skills needed to induce lactation and to give the mother confidence in her ability to do so on a day-to-day basis. She will also need support from her family and friends so that the process is not undermined. Putting her in contact with other mothers who have relactated or induced lactation may be helpful.

Before induced lactation commences, a full history must be taken as to why the mother had a poor milk supply or why she discontinued breastfeeding, in order to ensure that there are no factors that may continue to inhibit milk production, such as prolonged separation from the infant, supplementary feeding, use of teats/dummies, smoking, the combined contraceptive pill or medical reasons. Once the reason is identified this must be rectified, where possible, before continuing the process.

The process of induced lactation

The WHO (1998b) suggests there are two essential requirements for inducing lactation: 'a strong desire by the mother or foster mother to feed the infant, and stimulation of the nipple'.

Maximum stimulation of the nipple and breast can be achieved by the following techniques:

- There should be long periods of uninterrupted skin-to-skin contact and access to the breast. Co-bathing is one way of providing a comfortable and relaxing environment.
- Position and attachment should be retaught, along with recognising feeding cues.
- Breastfeed and/or express milk 8–12 times per day. Include night times when there is an increased production of prolactin.
- Practice breast compression if the milk flow is slow.
- Avoid artificial teats and dummies.
- Use of a breastfeeding supplementer (see Chapter 8) during breastfeeding may encourage the infant to suckle when the milk supply is poor.

While the mother is establishing her milk supply it is important that the infant's nutritional needs are met. If expressed breastmilk is available, this should be given following a breastfeed; however, this may not be available for all infants and they may require formula milk. As it is important to avoid teats, this can be given by cup or spoon. The infant should be closely observed to ensure its nutritional needs are being met by assessing wet nappies and stool as well as weight gain.

If the above methods are not effective, pharmacological methods (galactagogues such as domperidone or metoclopramide) or herbal remedies (such as fenugreek, garlic or fennel) may be tried, but further research is required to assess their effectiveness when milk production has ceased altogether (WHO, 1998b).

Concluding comments

Professional, social and peer support is an important element in providing mothers with help and information to enable them to continue to breastfeed for as long as they want to. UNICEF BFI supports this and recommends that healthcare professionals 'identify sources of national and local support for breastfeeding and refer mothers to these prior to discharge from hospital' (2010e, p. 21); and Point 7 also recommends continued cooperation between healthcare staff, breastfeeding support groups and the local community.

To ensure community support is effective, healthcare professionals must be educated and develop the knowledge and skills required to be able to support and advise mothers with practical and useful information as well as provide evidence-based information for fathers, family and friends. How they develop this knowledge and skill will be the focus of the following chapter.

Reflective questions

1 How do mothers in your area of practice know about the support groups available to them?
2 How is information disseminated to fathers, families and friends in your area of practice?
3 What follow-up mechanisms are in place for breastfeeding mothers in the community, to assist them to continue to breastfeed exclusively until their infants are six months old?

Resources

- HSE *Guide for New and Expectant Mothers Who Work*
  www.hse.gov.uk/pubns/indg373.pdf
- La Leche League
  www.laleche.org.uk
- NHS *Breastfeeding and Work*
  www.breastfeeding.nhs.uk/en/materialforclients/downloads/
  breastfeedingandwork.pdf
- UNICEF Baby Friendly Initiative
  www.babyfriendly.org.uk

Chapter 11 Developing knowledge and skills to support breastfeeding mothers

- Learning outcomes
- Informed choice
- Communication skills
- Learning about breastfeeding
- Concluding comments
- Reflective questions

In order to support and advise breastfeeding mothers effectively, it is essential that midwives, health visitors and other healthcare professionals have the knowledge and skills to do this. The Nursing and Midwifery Council (NMC, 2008) stipulates that nurses, midwives and health visitors provide a high standard of practice and care at all times by:

- Using the best available evidence:
  - You must deliver care based on the best available evidence or best practice.
  - You must ensure that any advice you give is evidence-based if you are suggesting healthcare products or services.

- Keeping your skills and knowledge up to date:
  - You must have the knowledge and skills for safe and effective practice.
  - You must keep your knowledge and skills up to date throughout your working life.
  - You must take part in appropriate learning and practice activities that maintain and develop your competence and performance.

This chapter discusses the essential skills required by healthcare professionals to enable them to provide mothers and their families with accurate information and skilled support, so that they can make informed choices, for example communication skills, reflective practice and evidence-based practice.

Learning outcomes

By the end of this chapter you will be able to:

- understand what influences mothers in their infant feeding choices;
- demonstrate effective communication and teaching skills;
- reflect on the knowledge and skills required to promote, protect and support breastfeeding and demonstrate how they can be achieved.

Mapping the UNICEF UK BFI educational outcomes

8   Be equipped to provide parents with accurate, evidence-based information about activities which may have an impact on breastfeeding.

Informed choice

To enable women to make informed choices about their care, healthcare professionals must 'provide accessible, evidence-based information in a balanced and non-judgemental manner and then respect whatever option is chosen' (Adamson, 2004, p. 587). This can sometimes be difficult for healthcare professionals, who are aware of the evidence to support breastfeeding and at times have difficulty understanding why mothers make the choices they do. Women often make their choices based on personal or vicarious experience (Dykes, 2003) and professionals must be able to understand and predict this.

Box 11.1 Breastfeeding myths

- A fifth of women aged between 16 and 24 years believe that breastfeeding would ruin the shape of their breasts or body.
- Almost all women believe that some women do not produce enough milk to be able to breastfeed.

Source: *Breastfeeding Awareness Week Survey* (DH, 2004a).

TABLE 11.1 Reasons for planning to use infant formula

Reason	Percentage
Did not like the idea of breastfeeding	32
Other people can feed the baby	25
Fed previous children with infant formula	21
Breastfed previous children and didn't get on with it	15
Can see how much the baby has had	5
Would be embarrassed to breastfeed	6
Expecting to return to work soon	3
Feeding with infant formula is less tiring	3
Medical reasons for not breastfeeding	6
Convenient/due to mother's lifestyle	13
Domestic reasons, coping with other children	6

Source: Bolling *et al.* (2007, p. 117).

Table 11.1 identifies the reasons mothers gave for planning to use formula instead of breastfeeding in the *Infant Feeding Survey 2005* (Bolling *et al.*, 2007). This evidence further highlights the important role of the healthcare practitioner in providing practical information about the benefits of breastfeeding in terms mothers can understand and in being able to answer any questions, thereby dispelling any myths.

However, despite being provided with information on the benefits of breastfeeding, many mothers will still choose to formula feed either immediately after birth or at some point later on. It is important that this decision is respected and mothers are given the support and advice to do this correctly and safely (see Chapter 8).

Communication skills

It is essential that healthcare professionals develop good communication skills to enable them to provide mothers with accurate and relevant information to empower them to breastfeed with confidence. Unfortunately, communication was identified as an area of potential deficit by the NMC (2007, 2009), and a generic skills statement was developed to support the existing NMC pre-registration proficiencies. Many mothers perceive healthcare professionals as too busy to spend time with them, and therefore it is important to provide a relaxed and unrushed atmosphere to encourage the physiology of lactation.

A good starting point is to consider what is meant by good communication skills, as this appears to have become a ubiquitous term in healthcare in recent years. The Department of Health describes it as:

> a process that involves a meaningful exchange between at least two people to convey facts, needs, opinions, thoughts, feelings or other information through both verbal and non-verbal means, including face to face exchanges and the written word.
>
> (2003a, p. 1)

Communication should not only be about the exchange or transfer of information but also about how it contributes to the therapeutic relationship – getting to know the mother and what she wants from the situation. Poor communication can lead to a mother experiencing a loss of control over her situation, stress, anxiety and sometimes misunderstanding or conflicting advice, which ultimately leads to lack of support. As discussed in Chapter 2, stress and anxiety can have a profound effect on the physiology of lactation and undermine a mother's confidence in her ability to breastfeed. The DH (2003a, p. 2) identified 11 benchmarks of good practice for communication between healthcare professionals, patients and carers, adding that effective interpersonal communication needs to be considered in the context of:

✔ fundamental values including openness, honesty and transparency;
✔ the importance of consent and confidentiality;
✔ the principles of common courtesy;
✔ self-awareness and the importance of body language and other non-verbal communication;
✔ skills such as establishing rapport, active and empathic listening, and being non-judgemental;
✔ the importance of using straightforward language and avoiding jargon;
✔ the need to adapt approaches to communication, and to be sensitive to language and cultural differences (using interpreters where appropriate), to individual developmental needs and disabilities (using aids and appliances as necessary) and to the psychological state and the experience of the mother and/or carer;
✔ the content of the communication and the situation, such as conveying bad news, dealing with complaints and resolving disputes and hostile situations.

To communicate effectively, particular attention needs to be paid to the person's hearing, vision and other physical and cognitive abilities, as well as to their preferred language and possible need for an interpreter.

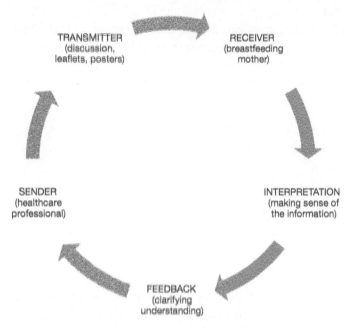

FIGURE 11.1 Communication processes: discussing breastfeeding

Communication of any message is a complex process and takes verbal, non-verbal and symbolic forms. For a message to be transferred effectively there must be a shared understanding of the content and structure of the message, which involves appreciation of attitudes, knowledge, social and cultural ideas that both the sender and receiver of the message possess. Often healthcare professionals assume that others understand professional terminology and abbreviations and take it for granted that they have prior understanding of the context of the message. A useful tool often used to explain the processes of communication in nursing and midwifery is based on Aristotle's theory of the requirements for effective communication – 'Speaker- Subject-Audience', which has been further developed by many writers such as Shannon and Weaver in 1949 and Berlo in the 1960s. (See Januszewski, 2001 for details of various communication models.) The model in Figure 11.1 is based on these ideas.

- **Sender**
  The sender is the person or persons (organisation) who begin the communication process and are responsible for encoding or translating the message. This may be influenced by the sender's attitude, knowledge and social and cultural experiences.

- **Transmitter**
  The content of the message is encoded or translated and structured using symbols such as language, literature, pictures or non-verbal cues etc. It is critical at this point that these symbols can be understood by the receiver for communication to be effective.

- **Receiver**
  The person receives the message through the senses, such as hearing, seeing, touching or tasting, and begins the process of decoding or interpretation.

- **Interpretation**
  Interpretation takes place using the same processes that the sender used to construct the message, attitude, knowledge and social and cultural experiences to make sense of the message.

- **Feedback**
  Berlo (1960) suggested that the communication process was incomplete until feedback from the receiver was received by the sender and the sender had in turn responded. The aim is to clarify that shared understanding has taken place.

Barriers to good communication

Between transmission and receiving there can be interference leading to misunderstanding, or the message is never received. This can be caused by the following:

- *Non-verbal cues*: negative body language – facial expressions, posture or poor eye contact.
- *Language*: technical terminology, too much information, language barriers, and level and tone of voice.
- *Attitude*: cultural and social norms, values and rules, pre-conceived ideas, prejudice and previous experience.
- *Individual aspects*: health and emotional status and cognitive skills.
- *Environment*: appropriateness to message – privacy, noise or distraction.

Lubbers (1990) suggested that the six most important skills for communication are:

- listening;
- relationship-building;
- instructing;

- motivation;
- exchanging information;
- giving feedback.

It could be argued that emotional intelligence could be added to this list. The main components of emotional intelligence are understanding yourself and understanding others through self-awareness, social awareness, self-management and social skills, all of which are essential for good communication processes.

It is important that women are given appropriate information to make informed choices. Part of this is ensuring that mothers receive unbiased information that is based on evidence. Every mother will perceive her breastfeeding experience differently and these experiences should not be undermined or judged by the healthcare professional. Nor should it be assumed that she has the knowledge she needs to breastfeed successfully even if she has had previous experience.

Step 5 of the *Ten Steps* recommends that all mothers should be given help with breastfeeding within six hours of giving birth, as well as being shown how to position and attach the infant at the breast, how to hand express and how to use a breast pump if separated from the infant (UNICEF, 2010e). The BFI suggests that:

> the key aim of teaching mothers is to give them information on the basic anatomy and physiology of breastfeeding and how to recognise effective attachment. That way if difficulties arise after the mother has left your care, she has some useful tools for helping her to solve [them].
>
> (UNICEF, 2008b, p. 38)

Activity

Reflect on a recent experience where you were trying to convey information to a breastfeeding mother.

- Did the communication process remain intact?
- Did she understand the message and give you feedback to clarify a shared understanding?
- If not, what do you think went wrong and how would you change things in the future?
- How did you gauge if the process was effective?

The principles recommended by the BFI (UNICEF, 2008a) to teach mothers are:

- Demonstrate techniques using appropriate visual aids.
- Give a rationale for what you are suggesting.
- Use a logical approach.
- Use appropriate language.
- Refer to principles that can be transferred to other situations.
- Build the mother's confidence so that she can help herself.

Learning about breastfeeding

As discussed in Chapter 1, the lack of knowledge and skills of healthcare professionals is a major contributing factor for poor breastfeeding rates (Renfrew *et al.*, 2005). So how do healthcare professionals learn about breastfeeding, and how do they develop a repertoire of skills and knowledge to promote, support and protect breastfeeding?

Breastfeeding knowledge and skills can be influenced by:

- research;
- clinical experience;
- trial and error;
- habitual practice ('the way things are done around here');
- personal experience, belief, values and attitudes;
- organisational issues.

Each of these factors is an important component in learning about breastfeeding and decision-making in practice, but in isolation can lead to conflicting advice and inappropriate care (Craig, 2002). Fawcett *et al.* (2001) support a holistic approach to learning, but also caution against exclusive emphasis on one method of acquiring knowledge such as research, and recommend an approach such as Carper's (1978) and White's (1995), to facilitate different ways of viewing and interpreting evidence to put into practice.

Carper (1978, p. 13) believed that, in order to teach and learn about nursing successfully, it was necessary to understand the 'patterns, forms and structure' of the body of knowledge that informs clinical practice. She described four fundamental patterns of knowing, which when used together would ensure nurses and midwives were equipped to provide appropriate, acceptable and holistic care for their clients. She emphasised that the components were interrelated and therefore each was dependent on the others.

- *Empirics, the science of nursing*: a systematic method of enquiry looking at care in an objective way; evidence-based practice. Carper believed that this was the first fundamental pattern of knowing.
- *Aesthetics, the art of nursing*: this is often misinterpreted as describing the psychomotor skills of practice. Instead, it refers to knowing that is subjective and unique, including creative approaches to care that are not always based on empirical evidence; it is perceiving the client as a whole and responding to their individual needs.
- *The component of personal knowledge*: this is sometimes confused with factual knowledge. However, Carper described personal knowledge as the most essential pattern of knowing, while being the most difficult to teach. Personal knowing is also subjective and is about learning to know ourselves, and using experience to develop effective interpersonal skills and learning to understand ourselves and how we relate to others.
- *Ethics, moral knowledge*: decision-making in clinical practice can be difficult because of the unique nature of individual clinical situations. Carper believed that ethical knowing is more than understanding codes and guidelines, and suggested that it included knowing what is right and wrong in the provision of care, particularly when making value judgements.

White (1995) added yet another pattern, 'socio-political', which she believed to be fundamental to all the other patterns. This additional pattern moves the focus from the individual relationship and situates it in a wider context, encouraging the nurse to examine professional practice and the politics of service provision. White (1995) related socio-political knowing to cultural identity and suggested that, in order to understand concepts of health, the nurse must have a wider knowledge of the social, political and economic influences on service provision. This pattern is crucial to knowing about breastfeeding and is demonstrated in the *Infant Feeding Survey 2005* (Bolling *et al.*, 2007), where patterns of social and cultural influences are evident in breastfeeding rates in the UK.

Reflective practice

Another way practitioners learn is through reflection. Schön (1983) highlighted reflection as a defining characteristic of a profession. Reflection and reflective practice have become ubiquitous terms in nursing and midwifery practice and are associated with deep learning, but the terms are sometimes confused.

Reflective practice is when practitioners learn through experience and, through the process of reflection, identify how they feel about the situation in light of current knowledge and are then able to plan for future action. Heath

(1998) suggested that, where problems are complex, reflection may assist nurses and midwives to develop a reasoned argument for a change in practice. Boud *et al.* (1985) claimed that structured reflection is key to learning from experience and described three stages students go through: preparation, engagement and processing, including reflective activity at each stage.

Schön (1983) divided the process of reflection into two categories: 'reflection-on-action' and 'reflection-in-action'. Reflection-on-action refers to the practice of thinking critically about an event after it has occurred, while reflection-in-action, which is usually only evident in the competent practitioner, occurs while carrying out a procedure or providing care, often unconsciously, but demonstrating that the practitioner is using creative approaches within individual situations.

There are many different models to aid the process of reflection and it is personal preference as to which is used. Gibbs' (1998) reflective cycle is commonly used by students due its simple but structured step-by-step approach.

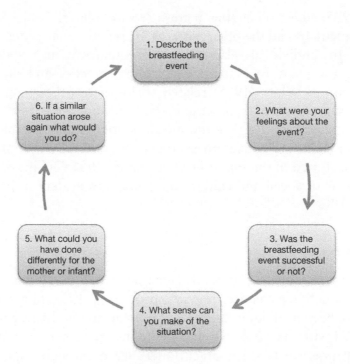

FIGURE 11.2 Reflecting on a breastfeeding event

Source: adapted from Gibbs (1998).

Reflection on parenthood education class using Gibbs' reflective cycle

Description Describe what happened during the breastfeeding event.

I had been asked to take a local parenthood education class for multiparous women in an area of high unemployment and deprivation to discuss breast-feeding. Breastfeeding rates in this area are low and I was aware that all the women had previously bottle-fed. I wanted to discuss the benefits of breastfeeding without causing any offence.

I explained about the research that has been carried out in relation to the benefits for mother and baby. I did not want anyone to feel guilty about their previous choice of infant feeding and tried to make the session quite light-hearted. Most of the women appeared receptive to the idea that breast was best, but one woman, Mrs B, was very confrontational, insisting that her previous child was healthy and that she and all her family had been bottle-fed and turned out all right and that breastfeeding was for middle-class women.

Feelings What were you thinking or feeling during the event?

Initially, I was very nervous that I would cause offence but felt confident in the information I was supplying. However, when Mrs B became confrontational and unwilling to take my message on board I felt very self-conscious and uncomfortable. I did not want to embarrass her, but had to continue and present the evidence to support breastfeeding and highlight the dangers inherent in bottle feeding.

Evaluation What went well or not so well in this event?

I had prepared well for the session using up to date evidence-based material to address the outcomes of the session that had been given to me by the person who normally takes the class. I had made a lesson plan and ensured that I kept to time. I felt the session was light hearted while getting the message across to most of the group. I introduced the topic, said what I was going to say, said it and then summed it up at the end. The other women appeared to listen.

However, Mrs B, was quite verbally aggressive and unwilling to listen or discuss the issues. My intention had been to provide the group with informa-tion that they may not have received before and also to get them to think about the possibility of breastfeeding and to support them to address the challenges they may face. Unfortunately Mrs B was quite disruptive and I found the session very challenging. I was embarrassed and found it difficult to reply to her statements.

Analysis What sense can you make out of the situation? Break it down into parts to explore in more detail.

The result of the session was that both Mrs B and myself left the session unsatisfied and that Mrs B had not taken in any of the information I had provided. I felt that I had been unable to deal with her confrontational attitude and that it had disrupted the session for the other women. I realise that it was not Mrs B's intention to be disruptive and that she probably felt I was attacking the choices she and her family had previously made.

I have discussed the episode with other clinicians and feel that I should have made the session more interactive, facilitating the discussion rather than just presenting information. For example, I could have done this by using the 'benefits of breastfeeding' poster as a visual aid to start the discussion about the benefits of breastfeeding for both mother and baby, and played clips from the DVD, *Best Beginnings: Bump to Breastfeeding*, to prompt further discussion. I could also have given each woman a locally produced leaflet to take home to discuss with her family.

Conclusion Now you have looked at it from different angles is there anything else you could have done or should not have done?

I realise that situations like this will always arise. It is probable that I took the wrong approach and could have presented the evidence in a more user-friendly and interactive way. Maybe the language I used was inappropriate, as was my presentation style, and Mrs B could have misinterpreted it and felt I was being condescending.

Action plan What would you do differently in a similar situation?

I feel more aware of the need to tailor the session for the client group and, instead of presenting information, I will make the session more interactive. The next time I conduct a session I will ask someone to attend with me for support and to give me some critical feedback.

TABLE 11.2 Summary of Johns' model of structured reflection (1995) in relation to Carper's (1978) four patterns of knowing

Carper's four patterns of knowing in nursing	Johns' cue questions for reflection
Empirics	What knowledge did or should have informed me?
Aesthetics	What was I trying to achieve? Why did I respond as I did? What were the consequences for the client? Others? Myself? How did the client feel? How did I know this?
Personal knowing	How did I feel in this situation? What internal factors were influencing me?
Ethics	How did my actions match with my beliefs? What factors made me act in incongruent ways?

Another commonly used model for reflection was developed by Johns, who compiled a set of questions based around Carper's (1978) four patterns of knowing (see Table 11.2) with the aim of encouraging the practitioner to be reflexive about their practice and adaptable to new situations. In contrast to Carper, Johns (1995) identified aesthetics to be at the root of knowing, and that the empirical, personal and ethical knowing all inform the holistic response to a clinical situation. He suggested that, in order to provide individualised care, the nurse must interpret the empirical evidence to suit the clinical situation rather than the other way around. Johns (1995) developed cue questions to aid practitioners to make sense of their experiences and to identify the areas of knowing that are required to provide effective, safe and satisfying care for clients.

The current focus on objective, empirical evidence, where randomised controlled trials are seen as the gold standard, has led to concerns that nurses and midwives may not be able to respond fully to the complex and diverse nature of clinical situations with which they are faced. Paley *et al.* (2007) conducted a comprehensive literature review to compare nursing's patterns of knowing with those of cognitive science, establishing that scientific knowledge still had priority over other forms of knowledge. However, for care to be meaningful and effective, objective empirical knowledge cannot be exclusive. It cannot provide the answers to all practice questions and needs to be considered alongside other forms of qualitative evidence as well as the other patterns of knowing (White, 1995).

Evidence-based practice

Evidence-based practice has also become a ubiquitous term in nursing and midwifery practice, but there is often confusion between the terms evidence-based practice, audit and research:

- Research is the systematic search to discover new information.
- Evidence-based practice uses the best available evidence to provide effective care.
- Audit is the process for reviewing care against best practice standards.

Evidence-based care is described as 'doing the right things right' (Gray, 2001) and 'the conscientious, explicit and judicious use of current best evidence in making decisions about the care of individual patients' (Sackett *et al.*, 1996, p. 71). However, to be effective it must take into account:

- clinical expertise;
- best available evidence;
- patient preference.

(Gray, 2001)

A variety of evidence can be used when deciding on the most appropriate line of care for mothers who are breastfeeding, but it must be assessed in conjunction with the individual event or situation, which will include psychosocial factors as well as physical ones. Healthcare professionals must be able to evaluate the strength of evidence identifying reliability, validity and generalisability; this is commonly done by rating research in a hierarchy of evidence (see Figure 11.3).

The Cochrane Library database contains regularly updated systematic reviews prepared by the Cochrane Collaboration (www.cochrane.org). A systematic review can be described as a literature review of the available studies on a particular subject, which is then analysed and synthesised, resulting in an objective conclusion about the cost-effectiveness and appropriateness of interventions or treatments. If the results are inconclusive, the recommendation for research may be made (Parahoo, 2006). Hemingway (2009) describes the processes involved in undertaking a systematic review as:

1 defining the appropriate question;
2 searching the literature;
3 assessing the studies;
4 combining the results;
5 placing the findings in context.

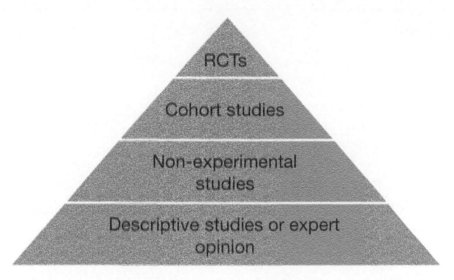

(RCTs = Randomised Controlled Trials)

FIGURE 11.3 The hierarchy of evidence

The aim of systematic reviews is to remove errors of interpretation and bias. Any misleading information and unsupported opinions are also likely to be removed. However, not all breastfeeding problems are capable of being solved by scientific means, resulting in limited available evidence. Evidence-based practice may offer some solutions and suggest a way forward, but it is not an answer for all the situations that professionals may encounter and therefore can limit the choice for both the expert and the mother, as the professional cannot justify using non-researched practices. This is evident throughout this book, where evidence is limited in support of some areas of practice. An example of a systematic review used throughout this book to support interventions to promote breastfeeding is taken from Renfrew *et al.* (2005), *The Effectiveness of Public Health Interventions to Promote the Duration of Breastfeeding: Systematic review*, which was commissioned by the Health Development Agency. Other useful sources of breastfeeding information can be found later in this chapter in the section 'Finding the evidence' and resources specific to breastfeeding can be found at the end of each chapter.

Healthcare professionals must not rely on systematic reviews alone and need to learn critical appraisal skills themselves. All graduate programmes now include a module on research, which includes how to critically review literature and appraise evidence-based practice. Critical appraisal skills are essentially the skills required to read research papers and make decisions about their reliability, validity and generalisability of evidence.

Activity

There are a number of issues you might wish to consider in relation to your place of study or work.

- Do you know how to access online databases and journals?
- Can you search for, and find, the appropriate literature to answer your questions adequately?
- Do you have the appropriate skills and knowledge to make judgements about the evidence you collect?

If you are having problems with any of these areas, make an appointment with your subject librarian who will be happy to help you.

Clinical guidelines and policies are based on the best available evidence at the time. Walsh and Wiggens describe this as translating the evidence for use in practice in 'useable, useful and relevant ways' (2003, p. 33). These can be national guidelines such as those published by NICE, or locally developed guidance as is required for Step 1/Point 1 of the BFI standards: 'Have a written policy that is routinely communicated to all staff'. Clinical guidelines are usually presented as detailed protocols, clinical pathways for groups of patients or algorithms to aid decision-making.

Finding the evidence

It is important to know where to look for evidence and to be able to access it. In recent years there have been a number of online developments in this area for healthcare professionals. Below are some useful sites you can access. Remember to use librarians to help you as they have a wealth of information and are happy to help you to improve your ability to search for literature.

- *The Cochrane Database of Systematic Reviews* contains regularly updated systematic reviews prepared by the Cochrane Collaboration: www. cochrane.org.
- *The Department of Health (DH)* aims to improve the health and well-being of the public: www.dh.gov.uk/en/index.htm.
- *The National Institute for Health and Clinical Excellence (NICE)* is an independent organisation responsible for providing national guidance on promoting good health and preventing and treating ill health: www. nice.org.uk.

- *The National Library for Health* is a gateway to many sources of health information for healthcare professionals: www.library.nhs.uk.
- *NIdirect* provides information on Northern Ireland policies. It has a useful publications section for accessing policy documents: www.nidirect.gov.uk.
- *Northern Ireland's HSC Public Health Agency*: http://publichealth.hscni.net.
- *The Nursing and Midwifery Council (NMC)* provides access to publications and policies relevant to nursing and professional practice: www.nmc-uk.org.
- *The Royal College of Midwifery (RCM)* provides access to online journals and has related evidence on professional issues: www.rcm.org.uk.
- *The Royal College of Nursing (RCN)* provides access to online journals and has related evidence on professional issues: www.rcn.org.uk.
- *Scotland's Health on the Web* has online health information provided by NHSScotland: www.show.scot.nhs.uk.
- *The Scottish Government* provides information on policies for Scotland. It has a useful publications section for accessing policy documents: www.scotland.gov.uk/home.
- *The Welsh Assembly Government* provides information on policies for Wales. It has a useful publications section for accessing policy documents: www.wales.gov.uk.
- *The World Health Organization (WHO)* is the directing and coordinating authority for health within the United Nations system. It is responsible for providing leadership on global health matters, shaping the health research agenda, setting norms and standards, articulating evidence-based policy options, providing technical support to countries and monitoring and assessing health trends: www.who.int.

Concluding comments

Communication skills are key to supporting mothers with breastfeeding and to provide them with information that they can understand and use, to help them continue breastfeeding for as long as they would like to. Doing this will empower mothers to make informed choices on the most appropriate care for them, their infants and their families. However, it must be remembered that, as there are numerous sources of information today, particularly from the internet, care must be taken to ensure that information is from reputable sources.

Reflective questions

1   Using your own choice of reflective model, reflect on a recent episode of care when supporting a mother with breastfeeding, where you can identify the use of Carper's four patterns of learning. Highlight where you obtained the evidence to support your practice and where it fits into the hierarchy of evidence.

2   Keep a reflective journal to provide evidence of your learning for your personal portfolio. This will enable you to organise your thoughts and encourage self-awareness and exploration of your actions or omissions in providing care for breastfeeding mothers.

Appendix 1

UNICEF UK Baby Friendly Initiative outcomes for higher education (updated 2008)

Basic knowledge and skills

1 Understand the importance of breastfeeding and the consequences of not breastfeeding in terms of health outcomes.

The education required to meet this learning outcome is as follows:

- The evidence-based health benefits, short and long term, of breastfeeding for mothers and babies.
- The risks associated with formula feeding, both full and partial.
- The differences between breastmilk and formula milk.
- The value of colostrum.
- Current recommendations regarding the duration of exclusive breast-feeding.

2 Have developed an in-depth knowledge of the physiology of lactation and be able to apply this in practical situations.

The education required to meet this learning outcome is as follows:

- External anatomy of the breast, normal variations of the size and shape of breast, nipple and areola.
- Relevant internal anatomy of the breast (with discussion of new evidence in this area).
- Normal changes in the breast during puberty, pregnancy and lactation.
- The role of the pituitary gland and the action of the lactational hormones, including their effects on behaviour.
- The prolactin receptor theory.
- The role of the feedback inhibitor of lactation (FIL) in the maintenance of lactation.
- The significance of the fat gradient of a breastfeed.
- The importance of early feeding/expression and frequent, effective drainage of the breast to ensure adequate ongoing milk production.

3   Be able to recognise effective positioning, attachment and suckling and to empower mothers to develop the skills necessary for them to achieve these for themselves.

The education required to meet this learning outcome is as follows:

- The difference between positioning and attachment.
- Definition and recognition of effective attachment and its importance for effective drainage of the breast.
- The mechanism of suckling, the suck/swallow cycle and recognition of effective feeding.
- The principles of positioning for breastfeeding and why these matter.
- Communication skills; effective teaching techniques, including identification of suitable resources (e.g. visual aids) for teaching positioning and attachment.

4   Be able to demonstrate knowledge of the principles of hand expression and have the ability to teach these to mothers.

The education required to meet this learning outcome is as follows:

- Why mothers should be enabled to learn hand expression of breastmilk.
- How hand expression differs from mechanical (pump) expression and reasons why it may be preferable.
- The technique of hand expression.
- Ways to assist the milk ejection reflex.
- Communication skills; effective teaching techniques, including identification of suitable resources (e.g. visual aids) for teaching hand expression.

Initiation and management of normal breastfeeding

5   Understand the potential impact of delivery room practices on the wellbeing of mother and baby and on the establishment of breastfeeding in particular.

The education required to meet this learning outcome is as follows:

- The innate reflexes, responses and abilities of the normal newborn baby.
- The physiological changes that occur at birth and the needs of the neonate for warmth, food and maternal contact.
- The role and importance of a period of unhurried skin contact between mother and baby at birth.
- The importance of breastfeeding as a means of promoting and assisting the adaptation of the infant to extrauterine life.

For midwifery students, the following are also essential:

- The impact of medications that may be used during labour on the condition and behaviour of the neonate.
- The role of the midwife in facilitating early mother–infant interaction and breastfeeding.
- The role of the midwife in ensuring the safety and well-being of the mother and baby in the immediate postnatal period.

6 Understand why it is important for mothers to keep their babies near them.

The education required to meet this learning outcome is as follows:

- The benefits of mothers keeping their babies near for early recognition of the infant's feeding cues and therefore for demand feeding.
- The relevance of mothers keeping their babies near for the prevention of infection.
- The relevance of mothers keeping their babies near in the prevention of sudden infant death syndrome.
- The information that must be shared with parents to enable informed decisions and safe practice around adult–infant bed sharing.

7 Understand the principle of demand feeding and be able to explain its importance in relation to the establishment and maintenance of lactation.

The education required to meet this learning outcome is as follows:

- The principle of supply and demand and its importance in promoting and ensuring adequate breastmilk supply.
- The nature and recognition of infant feeding cues.
- The importance of explaining demand feeding to parents.

8 Be equipped to provide parents with accurate, evidence-based information about activities that may have an impact on breastfeeding.

The education required to meet this learning outcomes is as follows:

- The nature and basis of different attitudes to breasts and breastfeeding and of how these may be influenced.
- The potential impact of mother–infant separation, restricted feeding practices, supplementation and the use of teats and dummies on breast-feeding and infant health.
- The definition and importance of informed choice.
- Communication skills, including the importance of giving full, unbiased information in a non-judgemental way.

Beyond the newborn period

9 Understand the importance of exclusive breastfeeding for the first six months of life and possess the knowledge and skills to enable mothers to achieve this.

The education required to meet this learning outcome is as follows:

- The reasons for the current recommendations regarding the duration of exclusive breastfeeding.
- The impact of supplementary feeds on successful breastfeeding.
- The common situations that lead to the introduction of supplementary feeds and how these may be avoided.
- The incremental benefits associated with how exclusively and for how long breastfeeding is practised.
- The importance of getting breastfeeding off to a good start.

10 Understand the importance of timely introduction of complementary foods and of continuing breastfeeding during the weaning period, into the second year of life and beyond.

The education required to meet this learning outcome is as follows:

- The reasons for the current recommendations regarding the appropriate age for the introduction of solid food.
- The value of longer-term breastfeeding to the health and well-being of both mother and baby.

For health visiting/public health nursing students, the following are also essential:

- Recognition of developmental readiness for solid feeding.
- When and how to introduce solid foods.

11 Understand the importance of community support for breastfeeding and demonstrate an awareness of the role of community-based support networks, both in supporting women to breastfeed and as a resource for health professionals.

The education required to meet this learning outcome is as follows:

- The importance of support for women in enabling both initiation and continuation of breastfeeding.
- The existing sources of support for breastfeeding families, both professional and voluntary, and how to access them.

- The role of voluntary sector breastfeeding counsellors/supporters.
- The role and value of support groups and peer support schemes.
- The importance of effective communication and handover of care between agencies (e.g. between midwife and health visitor).

Special situations and common complications

12 Be able to support mothers who are separated from their babies (e.g. on admission to SCBU, when returning to work) to initiate and/or maintain their lactation and to feed their babies optimally.

The education required to meet this learning outcome is as follows:

When separation occurs from birth:

- The importance of breastmilk for all babies, including those who are preterm, ill or compromised.
- The importance of early breastmilk expression in initiating and establishing lactation.
- How to optimise lactation through frequent expression, breast 'switching', dual expression.
- The value of skin contact/kangaroo mother care for the baby's well-being and for stimulating lactation and mothering.
- The unique role of hand expression in the first few days.

Ongoing care and later separation:

- The importance of frequent, effective breastmilk expression in maintaining breastmilk production.
- The value of skin contact whenever mother and baby are together.
- Methods of stimulating/assisting the let-down reflex.
- The ongoing value of hand expression and the appropriate use of breast pumps.
- Ways to help mothers re-establish/induce lactation.
- Storage of breastmilk, both for home use and for baby in SCBU.

13 Be able to demonstrate a knowledge of alternative methods of infant feeding and care which may be used where breastfeeding is not possible and which will enhance the likelihood of a later transition to breastfeeding.

The education required to meet this learning outcome is as follows:

- The alternative feeding methods available when babies are unable to breastfeed.

- The benefits and risks of alternative feeding methods.
- How to feed a baby safely using these methods.
- The benefits of skin-to-skin contact during feeding.

14 Identify babies who require a managed approach to feeding and describe appropriate care.

The education required to meet this learning outcome is as follows:

- Identification and appropriate management of babies who cannot demand feed (e.g. premature, small for gestational age, infected).
- Recognition and appropriate (pro-active) management of healthy, term newborns who are reluctant to feed.
- Recognition and management of the baby who is not receiving an adequate breastmilk intake.
- The management of neonatal jaundice in the breast-fed baby.
- Acceptable clinical indications for supplementation.
- The prevention and management of breast refusal.

For midwifery students, the following are also essential:

- The definition, diagnosis, prevention and management of neonatal hypoglycaemia.
- The management of the breast-fed baby of a diabetic mother.

15 Know about the common complications of breastfeeding, how these arise and how women may be helped to overcome them.

The education required to meet this learning outcome is as follows:

- The normal appearance of the lactating breast. Aetiology, recognition and appropriate management of nipple trauma, blocked duct, engorgement, mastitis and candida infection.
- Diagnosis and management of insufficient milk production in the mother.
- Ways to help mothers to re-establish or induce lactation, including managing supplementary feeding.

16 Understand the limited number of situations in which exclusive breastfeeding is not possible and be able to support mothers in partial breastfeeding or artificial feeding in these circumstances.

The education required to meet this learning outcome is as follows:

- The few, rare conditions of the mother and/or infant in which breastfeeding is contraindicated.

- The safe preparation and feeding of infant formula.
- The importance of practices such as skin-to-skin contact and rooming-in and demand feeding for all babies.

The Baby Friendly Initiative and the International Code

17 Appreciate the main differences between the WHO *International Code of Marketing of Breast-milk Substitutes* and the relevant current UK legislation and understand the relevance of the Code to their own work situation.

The education required to meet this learning outcome is as follows:

- Explanation of the Code and the UK law in relation to the advertising of breastmilk substitutes, bottles, teats and dummies.
- Key stipulations of the Code.
- How to ensure that the practices of individual healthcare staff and the workplace environment are in line with the Code.

18 Be thoroughly conversant with the Baby Friendly Initiative best practice standards, understand the rationale behind them and what the Baby Friendly Initiative seeks to achieve through them and be equipped to implement them in their own workplace, with appropriate support from colleagues.

The education required to meet this learning outcome is as follows:

- How the *Ten Steps/Seven Points* work together to enable women to initiate and maintain breastfeeding.
- The background to the BFI and its value as an accreditation scheme.
- Evidence for the effectiveness of the BFI as a public health intervention.
- The importance of being fully acquainted with the individual workplace's breastfeeding policy.
- The student's individual role and responsibility in implementing best practice related to breastfeeding.

Appendix 2

Nursing and Midwifery Council Essential Skills Clusters (ESCs) for pre-registration midwifery education

4: Initiation and continuance of breastfeeding

(Note: (BFI) = relates to Baby Friendly Initiative educational outcomes.)

Women can trust/expect a newly registered midwife to:	By the first progression point	For entry to the register
1. **Understand and share information that is clear, accurate and meaningful at a level which women, their partners and family can understand.**	Participates in communicating sensitively the importance of breastfeeding and the consequences of not breastfeeding, in terms of health outcomes (BFI). Observes a variety of forums where information is shared in respect of the advantages and disadvantages of different infant feeding methods.	Listens to, watches for and responds to verbal and non verbal cues. Uses skills of being attentive, open-ended questioning and paraphrasing to support information sharing with women. Able to lead a variety of forums where information is shared with women about the advantages and disadvantages of different infant feeding methods, without regarding breastfeeding and artificial feeding as 'equal' choices. Understands the importance of exclusive breastfeeding and the consequences of offering artificial milk to breastfed babies. Critically appraises the nature and strength of breastfeeding promotional and support interventions. Understands the nature of evidence and how to

Women can trust/expect a newly registered midwife to:	By the first progression point	For entry to the register
		evaluate the strength of research evidence used to back information.
		Keeps accurate records of the woman and her baby relating to breastfeeding, including plans of care and any problems encountered or referrals made.
2. Respect social and cultural factors that may influence the decision to breastfeed.	Has an awareness of own thoughts and feelings about infant feeding in order to facilitate information sharing to be ethical and non-judgemental.	Demonstrates a working knowledge of the local demographic area and explores strategies to support breastfeeding initiatives within the locality.
	Is sensitive to issues of diversity when sharing information with women. Skilfully explores attitudes to breastfeeding.	Respects the rights of women.
		Takes into account differing cultural traditions, beliefs and professional ethics when communicating with women.
3. Effectively support women to breastfeed.	Willingness to learn from women.	Applies in-depth knowledge of the physiology of lactation to practice situations (BFI).
	Assists in ensuring that the needs of women are met in developing clear care pathways. Participates in explaining to women the importance of baby-led feeding in relation to the establishment and maintenance of breastfeeding (BFI).	Can recognise effective positioning, attachment, suckling and milk transfer.
		Uses skills of observation, active listening and on-going critical appraisal in order to analyse the effectiveness of breastfeeding practices.
	Can recognise effective positioning, attachment, suckling and milk transfer.	Is confident at exploring with women the potential impact of delivery room practices, such as the effect of different pain relief methods and the importance of skin-to-skin contact, on the well-being of their baby and
	Is able to help teach mothers the necessary skills to enable them to effectively position and attach their baby for breastfeeding (BFI).	

213

Women can trust/expect a newly registered midwife to:	By the first progression point	For entry to the register
	Explains to women the importance of their baby rooming-in with them and baby holding in the postnatal period as a means of facilitating breastfeeding (BFI).	themselves and on the establishment of breastfeeding in particular (BFI).
	Recognises common complications of breastfeeding, how these arise and demonstrates how women may be helped to avoid them (BFI).	Uses appropriate skills to support women to be successful at breastfeeding for the first six months of life (BFI).
	Participates in teaching women how to hand express their breastmilk and how to store, freeze and warm it with consideration to aspects of infection control (BFI).	Explores with women the evidence base underpinning information, which may have an impact on breastfeeding, such as bed sharing and the use of dummies (BFI).
		Empowers women to recognise effective positioning, attachment, suckling and milk transfer for themselves (BFI).
		Is skilled at advising women over the telephone when contacted for advice on breastfeeding issues.
4. Recognise appropriate infant growth and development, including where referral for further advice/action is required.	Participates in assessing appropriate growth and development of the neonate.	Acts upon the need to refer when there is a deviation from appropriate infant growth.
	Participates in carrying out physical examinations as necessary, with parent's consent.	Demonstrates skills to empower women to recognise appropriate infant growth and development and to seek advice when they have concerns.
	Informs women of the findings from any assessment/examination performed, in a manner that is understood by the women.	
5. Work collaboratively with other practitioners and external agencies.	Works within the NMC *Code of Professional Conduct: Standards for conduct, performance and ethics.*	Practices within the limitations of their own competences, knowledge and sphere of professional practice, consistent with

Women can trust/expect a newly registered midwife to:	By the first progression point	For entry to the register
	Actively works as a team member.	the legislation relating to midwifery practice.
	Values others' roles and responsibilities in supporting women to breastfeed.	Works confidently, collaboratively and in partnership with women and others to ensure the needs of women are met.
	Shares information about national and local agencies and networks that are available to support women in the continuation of breastfeeding, such as Lactation Consultants, National Childbirth Trust and La Leche League for example.	Understands the importance of community support for breastfeeding and actively refers women to community-based support networks, both in supporting women to breastfeed and as a resource for health professionals (BFI).
		Actively works with other health professionals and external agencies to promote breastfeeding and support women in their choice to breastfeed.
		Is able to discuss with women the importance of exclusive breastfeeding for six months and timely introduction of complementary foods and continuing breastfeeding during the weaning period, into the second year of life and beyond.
6. Support women to breastfeed in challenging circumstances.	Is aware of the limited number of situations in which exclusive breastfeeding is not possible and participates in supporting women to partially breastfeed or artificially feed (BFI). Is sensitive to the needs of women and their partners.	Involves appropriate help, such as a lactation consultant, where specialised skills are required, in order to support women to successfully breastfeed. Acts upon the need to refer to appropriate health professionals where deviation from appropriate infant feeding and growth patterns is apparent.

Women can trust/expect a newly registered midwife to:	By the first progression point	For entry to the register
		Supports women who are separated from their babies (on admission to SCBU, women receiving high dependency care in a separate environment) to initiate and maintain their lactation and feed their babies optimally (BFI).
		Feeds expressed breastmilk to a baby, using a cup and/or syringe as appropriate (BFI).
		Teaches women how to use mechanical breast pump where appropriate.

Appendix 3

The *Ten Steps* and the *Seven Point Plan*

The *Ten Steps* (UNICEF UK BFI)

Step 1 Have a written breastfeeding policy that is routinely communicated to all health care staff.

Step 2 Train all health care staff in skills necessary to implement the policy.

Step 3 Inform all pregnant women about the benefits and management of breastfeeding.

Step 4 Help mothers initiate breastfeeding soon after birth.

Step 5 Show mothers how to breastfeed and how to maintain lactation, even if they should be separated from their infants.

Step 6 Give newborn infants no food or drink other than breastmilk, unless medically indicated.

Step 7 Practise rooming-in – allow mothers and infants to remain together 24 hours a day.

Step 8 Encourage breastfeeding on demand.

Step 9 Give no artificial teats or dummies to breastfeeding infants.

Step 10 Foster the establishment of breastfeeding support groups and refer mothers to them on discharge from hospital.

The *Seven Point Plan* for the Protection, Promotion and Support of Breastfeeding

Point 1 Have a written breastfeeding policy that is routinely communicated to all healthcare staff.

Point 2 Train all healthcare staff involved in the care of mothers and babies in the skills necessary to implement the policy.

Point 3 Inform all pregnant women about the benefits and management of breastfeeding.

Point 4 Support mothers to initiate and maintain breastfeeding.

Point 5 Encourage exclusive and continued breastfeeding, with appropriately timed introduction of complementary foods.

Point 6 Provide a welcoming atmosphere for breastfeeding families.

Point 7 Promote cooperation between healthcare staff, breastfeeding support groups and the local community.

For further details go to www.babyfriendly.org.uk.

Appendix 4
Lactation history

Mother's name: _____

Baby's name: _____

Date of birth: _____

Baby's age in months: _____

Reason for consultation: _____

1. Current feeding situation

Breastfeeds

- Approximate number of feeds in 24 hours: ....
- Average length of feeds: ....
- Longest gap between feeds: ....
- One breast or both breasts? ....

Supplements (if any)

- What: ....
  (formula/water/other drinks/solid foods)
- Frequency and quantity: ....
- Age when started: ....
- At whose suggestion? ....
- How given: ....
  (bottle/cup/other)

Dummy (if any)

- How often used and for how long at a time: ....
- Age when started: ....
- At whose suggestion? ....

Milk expression (if any)

- Frequency of expression: ....
- Quantities obtained: ....

Separation of mother and baby

- Where does baby sleep? ....
  By day: ....
  At night: ....
- Hours mother away from baby (e.g. at work): ....

2. Baby's current health and behaviour

Feeding behaviour

- Does baby demand feeds? ....
- Behaviour during feeds: ....
- Any vomiting? ....

General health

- Urine output: ....
  (frequency/colour)
- Stools: ....
  (frequency/colour/consistency)
- Weight: ....
  Centile: ....
- Length: ....
  Centile: ....
- Head circumference: ....
  Centile: ....
- Illnesses to date: ....
- Any abnormalities? ....
- Mother's feelings about baby's health and behaviour: ....

3. The early postnatal period

Baby's condition at birth

- APGAR score
  at 1 min: ....
  at 5 mins: ....
  at 10 mins: ....

- Weight: ....
  Centile: ....
- Length: ....
  Centile: ....
- Head circumference: ....
  Centile: ....

Early postnatal care

- Skin-to-skin contact began at: .... mins
  Duration: ....
- Reason for ending (or why not possible): ....
- Age at first breastfeed: ....
- Rooming-in? ....
  If not, why not? ....
- Details of any prelacteal feeds or supplements: ....
  (when/what/how given)
- Mother's experience of the early postnatal period: ....

4. Pregnancy and birth

Pregnancy

- Duration of pregnancy (i.e. gestation at birth): ....
- Multiple pregnancy? ....
- Progress of pregnancy: ....
- Breastfeeding discussed? ....
- Mother's experience of pregnancy: ....

Labour and delivery

- Nature of labour: ....
  (normal/induced/augmented)
- Type of delivery: ....
- Anaesthesia/analgesia (if any): ....
- Estimated blood loss: ....
- Placenta intact? ....
- Mother's experience of labour and delivery: ....

5. Mother's health

- Age: ....
- First language: ....

- Disabilities: ....
- Allergies/dietary needs: ....
- Health and medication history: ....
- Current health: ....
- Current medication: ....
  (caffeine consumption? ....)
- Current family planning method: ....
- Smoker? ....
- Alcohol consumption: ....

6. Previous infant feeding experience

- Number and ages of previous babies: ....
- How many breastfed: ....
- Nature of breastfeeding experience: ....
  (complications/supplements)
- Mother's feelings about these experiences: ....

7. Family and social situation

- Household consists of: ....
  (other family members)
- Financial concerns (if any): ....
- Mother working/intending to return to work? ....
- Mother's occupation: ....
- Working hours: ....
- Support from partner for breastfeeding: ....
- Support from other family members for breastfeeding: ....
- Help with child care: ....
- Mother's feelings about her situation: ....

Source: UNICEF (2008a, pp. 76–8).

Appendix 5

UNICEF UK BFI *Best Practice Standards for Establishing and Maintaining Lactation and Breastfeeding in Neonatal Units*

1. **Have a written (neonatal unit) breastfeeding policy which is routinely communicated to all staff**

- The neonatal unit should have a written breastfeeding policy which addresses all these standards and protects breastfeeding. The policy should be formulated in conjunction with the maternity and community services (where relevant) in order to ensure a seamless delivery of care. It should identify clearly the professional groups which will act as the point of first referral to support mothers to breastfeed.
- A summary of the policy should be prominently displayed in the unit. The full policy and any supporting guidance should be available on request. The policy and summary should be translated into other languages where appropriate. All neonatal unit managers should be able to easily locate a copy of the policy and be able to describe the process of staff orientation to the policy.
- Compliance with the policy should be audited annually and the results of this audit used to ensure continuing full implementation of all standards. Breastmilk feeding and breastfeeding rates on discharge from the unit should be recorded and progress reported to all staff.
- All policies and procedures should support breastmilk feeding and the establishment of breastfeeding in line with these standards.

2. **Educate all health care staff in the skills necessary to implement the policy**

- All health care staff should receive orientation to both the breastfeeding policy and any supporting guidance as soon as their employment on the neonatal unit begins.
- Education programmes which cover all of the standards will be provided for each professional group and area of responsibility.* Clear curricula or

course outlines for each group should be developed. A training schedule for new employees should exist.

- All staff caring for mothers and their babies should have received breast-feeding training appropriate to their role or, if new, have received orientation on arrival and be scheduled to receive training within six months.

It is recommended that the training for staff who have primary responsibility for supporting mothers to initiate and maintain lactation have at least 18 hours' breastfeeding education including a minimum of three hours' supervised practical skills review relating to teaching a mother how to breastfeed and how to hand express breastmilk.

3. **Inform all parents of the benefits of breastmilk and breastfeeding for babies in the neonatal unit**

- All parents whose baby is admitted, or is likely to be admitted, to the neonatal unit should have a one-to-one discussion with a suitably qualified* health professional about the crucial importance of breastmilk to the preterm and ill infant.** This discussion along with the parents' decision should be documented in the baby's records.
- Written materials provided to parents on the benefits of breastmilk and breastfeeding should be accurate and effective.

Suitably qualified health professionals would include paediatricians, infant feeding specialists, midwives and nurses who have been appropriately educated in breastfeeding and lactation management.

**The discussion on the importance of breastfeeding should emphasise the particular importance of breastmilk to the preterm and ill infant and will need to include information about the importance of breastmilk in relation to the prevention of necrotising enterocolitis and improvement of neurological development. The longer-term benefits of breastfeeding to babies and mothers should also be explained.*

4. **Facilitate skin-to-skin contact (kangaroo care) between mother and baby**

- The benefits of skin-to-skin contact should be discussed with all parents at an appropriate time to allow informed decision making. Skin-to-skin contact between mother and baby should be initiated in an unhurried environment as soon as the baby's condition allows. Skin-to-skin contact should continue to be offered as often as possible (*at least on a daily basis*) or whenever the mother is available and the baby's condition allows.

5. **Support mothers to initiate and maintain lactation through expression of breastmilk**

*   All mothers with a baby on the neonatal unit should be encouraged to initiate lactation as soon after delivery as the mother's condition allows. All mothers whose babies cannot breastfeed or take full feeds from the breast should be taught how to express their milk by hand and by pump. Expression of breastmilk should be encouraged at least six to eight times in 24 hours, including at night. Emphasis should be on frequent expressing and the avoidance of long intervals between expressions.
*   Well-maintained equipment for the safe expression of breastmilk should be available at all times.
*   Facilities should be available to allow mothers to express breastmilk in comfort either near their baby or in private if preferred.
*   Local policies on the safe handling, storage and transportation of breastmilk should be developed in line with nationally agreed guidelines.
*   A system for the provision of breast pumps for home use should also be in place.

6. **Support mothers to establish and maintain breastfeeding**

*   All breastfeeding mothers should be offered help with a first breastfeed as soon their baby's condition permits. Breastfeeding mothers should receive information, help and support to achieve correct positioning and attachment.*
*   When the baby is not yet able to take a full feed from the breast, mothers should be encouraged to practise positioning techniques.
*   Parents should be given information on the importance of baby-led feeding (as soon as appropriate) for the continuation of breastfeeding. They should be taught to recognise feeding cues and be encouraged to use all available opportunities to initiate breastfeeds.
*   The unit should have a policy of open visiting for parents. Facilities for rooming-in should be available and where possible mothers and babies should be enabled to room-in together.**
*   All written materials on infant feeding provided for parents should be accurate and effective.

It is recognised that some mothers may not wish to breastfeed, but may decide to continue expressing breastmilk. In this circumstance the mothers should be supported to continue providing breastmilk and given an informed choice regarding the short and long term benefits to baby of feeding directly from the breast.

** It is recognised that rooming-in facilities may not be available within the neonatal unit. However, new mothers should at least be cared for in the same hospital as their baby. Where facilities are available, breastfeeding mothers should be encouraged to room-in with their baby in the neonatal unit.

7. Encourage exclusive breastmilk feeding

- No food or drink other than breastmilk should be given to a baby who is being breastfed or receiving breastmilk unless this is clinically indicated or the result of a fully informed parental decision.
- A mother's own breastmilk is the first choice for infant feeding. Where mother's own milk is not available the use of donor milk should be considered and where possible obtained.
- When mothers are separated from their babies, mechanisms should exist to enable the regular transportation of the mother's milk to the facility caring for the baby.
- All written guidelines and protocols should support exclusive breast-feeding.*
- No promotion for breastmilk substitutes, feeding bottles, teats or dummies, should be displayed or distributed to parents or staff in the facility.

* Protocols for conditions such as hypoglycaemia, jaundice requiring photo-therapy or slow weight gain should protect exclusive breastfeeding. If breastmilk fortifiers are used, protocols should be developed to ensure use is limited to clear clinical indication, for example for very low birthweight (less than 1500g) babies when a biochemical assessment indicates a need.

8. Avoid the use of teats or dummies for breastfed babies unless clinically indicated

- Babies who are unable to feed directly from the breast should be fed breastmilk by a method appropriate to the baby's developmental ability. Parents wishing to breastfeed who request that their baby be fed by teat must have the potential risks discussed and alternatives offered.
- Dummy use should be limited to when there is a clear clinical indication or fully informed parental choice.
- Skin-to-skin contact and breastfeeding should be promoted for comforting babies and relieving pain during minor procedures such as heel pricks.
- Feeding and comforting methods appropriate to the baby's condition, and with reference to the presence or absence of the parents at any given time, should be discussed with the parents. The discussion should be evidence-based and include all potential benefits, risks and alternatives to allow

informed decision making. The discussion and the parents' choice should be recorded in the baby's notes or care plan.

9. Promote breastfeeding support through local and national networks

- All mothers should be provided with the contact details of midwives, health visitors, community neonatal nurses (where these exist), breastfeeding support networks and organisations which support parents of ill and premature babies for help with breastfeeding on admission to a neonatal unit and on discharge of the baby from hospital.
- A formal mechanism should exist to ensure that information on breast-feeding progress is passed on during handover of care from the neonatal unit to the community health care team.

Appendix 6
Milk banks in the UK

- **Birmingham**
  Birmingham Women's Health Care Trust, Metchley Park Road,
  Edgbaston
  Tel: 0121 472 1377

- **Cambridge**
  The Rosie Hospital
  Tel: 01223 217617

- **Cheshire**
  Countess of Chester Hospital, Liverpool Road, Chester
  Tel: 01244 366416

- **Co. Fermanagh**
  Unit 2, The Cornsheads, Mill Street, Irvinestown
  Tel: 028 686 28333

- **Glasgow**
  Yorkhill Donor Milk Bank, RPDU, Yorkhill
  Tel: 0141 201 0855

- **Huddersfield**
  Neonatal Unit, Claderdale Royal Hospital

- **Kent**
  NICU, Medway Maritime Hospital, Windmill Road, Gillingham
  Tel: 01634 825125

  Princess Royal University Hospital, Orpington
  Tel: 01689 864924

- **London**
  Guy's and St Thomas' NHS Foundation Trust, Lambeth Palace Road
  Tel: 020 7188 4030

King's College Hospital, Golden Jubilee Wing, King's College Hospital, Denmark Hill, Camberwell
Tel: 020 7346 3038

Kingston Hospital, Galsworthy Road, Kingston Upon Thames
Tel: 020 8974 5390

Queen Charlotte's and Chelsea Hospital, The Milk Bank Unit, Du Cane Road
Tel: 020 8383 3559

St George's Hospital, Blackshaw Road, Tooting
Tel: 020 875 1936

- **Oxford**
  John Radcliffe Hospital
  Tel: 01865 222076

- **Southampton**
  Princess Ann Hospital, Oxford Road
  Tel: 023 8079 6009

- **Surrey**
  St Peter's Hospital Milk Bank, NICU St Peter's Hospital, Guildford Road, Chertsey
  Tel: 01932 722667

- **Wirral**
  The Wirral Mothers' Milk Bank, Clatterbridge Hospital, Bebington
  Tel: 0151 334 4000

Answers to quizzes and scenarios

Chapter 2

True or false quiz

1 *False* The size of the breast is determined by the amount of fatty tissue. This does not predict milk storage capacity.

2 *True* Storage capacity is variable but over a 24-hour period all lactating mothers produce approximately 798g. Those with lower storage capacity will feed more frequently than their counterparts.

3 *True* Ramsay claimed the lactiferous ducts branch off within the areola and found no evidence of lactiferous sinuses.

4 *False* Geddes claims mothers can have multiple milk ejections during a feed ranging from 0–9.

5 *False* Water makes up about 80 per cent of milk volume and therefore infants do not need supplements. Supplements will interfere with milk production.

6 *True* Colostrum has a purgative effect on the bowel and helps clear meconium.

7 *True* As the feed progresses the fat level gradually increases.

8 *False* Secretory immunoglobulin A (sIgA), entero- and broncho-mammary pathways, white blood cells, and antibodies from previous maternal infections cannot be replicated in formula milk.

9 *True* Prolactin is inhibited until the delivery of the placenta and membranes (complete), resulting in decreased levels of progesterone, oestrogen, HPL and PIF.

10 *False* A build-up of FIL will decrease milk production and therefore the breasts should be emptied on a regular basis.

Chapter 3

Quiz

1 Sustainable position; head and neck in a straight line; allow infant to move its head freely; hold the infant close; nose to nipple; lead with the chin.
2 The underarm position.
3 Wide mouth; chin indents the breast; lower lip curled out; full cheeks; hear swallowing; see milk at the mouth; more areola at top than bottom.
4 Cheeks drawn in; both lips flanged; long or short feeds with an unsettled infant; explosive, watery, frothy stool; failure to thrive; nipple trauma; breast refusal.
5 At the end of the feed.
6 On day 5 to assess position and attachment and milk transfer.
7 Assess urine and stools and weight.
8 At least eight times, including night time when prolactin levels are high.
9 Wash hands and prepare storage equipment; comfortable position, massage breasts; feel around areola for difference in consistency; place thumb and first two fingers in a 'C' shape and gently compress at 6 and 12 o'clock about 2–3cms above the nipple; compress and release. As milk ejection ceases move to another position.
10 Increases prolactin levels and saves time.

Chapter 4

Scenario 1

• It is vital that Jane is aware of the many benefits offered by skin-to-skin contact for any age of infant. It will reduce crying in the baby and stabilise vital signs, and provide access to the breast.
• You could suggest co-bathing; this may well be very useful for Jane in settling the baby and having some relaxation in a bath too.
• Consider safe bed-sharing – provide Jane with the evidence relating to breastfeeding and SIDS and, if she makes the informed choice to take her baby into bed with her, explain the ways she can reduce the risk of accidents and overheating.

Scenario 2

- Obviously Joanne has been through a huge ordeal and is exhausted – she needs lots of positive feedback on how well she has done.
- Positioning and attachment have been described as 'good' – ask her to feed her baby again, giving her full support and encouragement. Observe a breastfeed for all the signs of effective positioning and attachment, as there may be a simple problem that has led to the situation of the baby feeding frequently.
- Is there family there who can cuddle the baby? If not, settle the baby beside her following the feed.
- Ask the paediatricians to review the baby and prescribe paracetamol – position the baby in a way so as not to lie on the affected side, if at all possible.
- Ensure that Joanne has effective analgesia and that her vital signs are all within normal limits.
- Maybe there are a lot of visitors and this may need to be monitored to ensure that Joanne is given time to recover.

Quiz

1 Sedated from maternal drugs in labour; undiagnosed illness; too hot/cold; feeding cues are missed; separated from mother.

2 Encourages breastfeeding; reduces crying; regulates temperature, respiratory rate and heart rate; promotes bonding.

3 Do not co-sleep on the sofa or bring the infant into bed if you smoke, have taken alcohol or drugs, or you or the infant are ill (preterm infants), or if you are extremely tired. Firm mattress; ensure infant cannot be trapped between you and the wall or fall out of bed; do not overdress the infant or leave it alone in bed; loose covers that do not go over the head; room temperature 16–18°C. No pets and if there is another child in the bed, ensure there is an adult between them and the infant.

4 Helps recognise feeding cues; facilitates unrestricted feeds; improves maternal confidence.

5 Reduces conflicting advice; ensures practice is consistent with WHO Code and UNICEF UK BFI standards; commitment from managers to implement good practice.

6 Posters, leaflets, verbal information.

7 To avoid using a dummy while establishing breastfeeding, particularly within the first month, because it may cause nipple confusion, reduce the number of feeds and decrease milk supply, and the mother is unable to

recognise feeding cues. It is also a potential portal for thrush and can lead to tooth decay and recurrent ear infections.

8 Demand feeding is feeding the infant when it shows signs of wanting to feed.

9 Supplementary feeds lead to reduced suckling and breast stimulation, reduced prolactin production, increased FIL and a decrease in milk supply.

10 Infant cues: sucking movements and noises, licking lips, head movements from side to side, rapid eye movement, restlessness. Crying is a late sign.

Chapter 5

Scenario 1

Determine the cause of the problem by taking a lactation history, examine Carmel's breasts and the infant's mouth for signs of any anomalies, and observe a complete breastfeed. Remind her to let the infant itself come off the breast and how to break the vacuum first if attachment is incorrect. Teach her the principles of position and attachment again and explain that, in order to maintain the milk supply, she also needs to continue to breastfeed or express from the affected side. Recommend different positions that she may find more comfortable. Because the skin is broken, moist wound healing is advisable.

Scenario 2

Remind Alison of the benefits of breastfeeding for herself and Eve. Take a lactation history and find out if she has support from family and friends to continue breastfeeding. Ask her for a history of the feeding pattern and if anything has changed, such as introducing a dummy or giving supplementary feeds. Determine if there is effective milk transfer by observing a breastfeed and assessing Eve's nappies and weight. Teach Alison the principles of position and attachment and how to assess milk transfer. Recommend she tries skin-to-skin contact and ensures that Eve is getting a full feed, receiving the fattier milk at the end of the feed.

Scenario 3

Determine the cause of the problem by taking a lactation history and observing a breastfeed. Inform Bridget that to maintain her milk supply she must breastfeed regularly from both sides and express following the feed to empty the breasts fully until the condition is resolved. If she is unable to feed from the affected side then she must express. If she does not do this it will make the situation worse. Advise her on changing position to aid drainage of the breast. Remind her about the principles of effective position and attachment and how to avoid blocked ducts. Recommend fluids and rest and advise her that she can take analgesia (ibuprofen and paracetamol). If the problem persists she may need antibiotics.

Chapter 6

Scenario

- Take a lactation history (see Chapter 5). Anne has several risk factors: large blood loss, blood transfusion, pain from her third-degree tear, long labour.
- Jonathan had a few risk factors for weight loss: he never had skin-to-skin initially, he had a cup feed of formula two hours after birth and then again eight hours after that.
- Observe a complete breastfeed for position and attachment and milk transfer.
- Reteach position and attachment and how to recognise feeding cues. Recommend that she avoid using teats and dummies.
- See Chapter 7 for managing weight loss, as this is 10 per cent loss.
- Encourage skin-to-skin contact.
- Anne should regularly feed Jonathan and frequently express to improve her supply of milk; this should include at least once at night.
- Plan to weigh regularly and observe milk transfer.

Chapter 7

Scenario 1

- Encourage skin-to-skin and rooming-in so Carol can pick up infant feeding cues.
- Encourage regular breastfeeds, at no more than three-hourly intervals, to increase bowel motility, clear meconium and reduce the reabsorption of unconjugated bilirubin. Advise Carol to wake Amy for feeds.
- Observe and assess breastfeeds to ensure adequate milk transfer.
- If the infant has difficulty feeding, weight loss is more than 7 per cent of the birthweight or there are signs of dehydration, Carol should be encouraged to express breastmilk following the feed and give this as a supplement or 'top-up' rather than formula and give it by cup rather than bottle.

Scenario 2

- Take a full breastfeeding history to discover if there is a feeding problem. Observe positioning and attachment to see if there may be a problem, for example with tongue-tie.
- Is there any history of thrush etc.?
- Has home life changed? Is Ingrid under stress? What other children does she have? Does she have a supportive family? What is her physical health like?
- Recommend skin-to-skin contact.
- Use a breast pump to increase lactation so that she can supplement the breastfeed and increase her milk supply and gradually reduce amounts of formula.
- Assess Gemma's nappies; are they wet, dirty? What colour is the stool?
- It may be useful to mention fenugreek and other remedies (if taking other medication discuss with GP).
- Close follow-up and reweighing over the next two weeks is very important.
- Use of a cup instead of a teat to supplement as necessary.

Chapter 9

Scenario

- Compliment Leasa on how well she has done with her exclusive breast-feeding and comment on how healthy Molly looks and that she is gaining weight beautifully.
- Reassure Leasa that Molly is just ensuring a good milk supply, that she may well be going through a growth spurt and that her breastmilk is all Molly will need for the first six months of life.
- Advise Leasa not to supplement with solids or formula. Molly is increasing her milk supply by feeding more frequently and stepping up milk production.
- Be understanding about the well-meaning relatives who have offered this advice, but remind Leasa about the problems that supplementing will have on her milk supply and the risk of triggering allergies and increasing the risk of childhood diabetes and obesity.
- Make sure nothing else has changed in Leasa's care of Molly. Has a dummy been introduced? Has she changed her sleeping arrangements?
- Remind Leasa about the signs of being ready to wean, for example reaching out to grab things, putting things to her mouth etc. If Molly is not demonstrating these traits, it may reassure Leasa that she is not ready to be weaned.

- Suggest taking Molly into bed to feed her if Leasa has to get up. Perhaps she could adapt her bed and cot to avoid unnecessary disruptions. See Chapter 4 for bed-sharing guidelines.
- If Leasa resents the interruptions to her sleep, she will face each day with frustration and will try harder and harder to fit her baby into her sleep pattern. However, if she adjusts her mental attitude to one of acceptance, she will find that she is able to enjoy those moments in the night when Molly needs to be nursed and comforted.

Glossary

Alveoli   Glands within the breast that produce milk. Tiny sacs that look like a bunch of grapes.

Aminoacidopathy   Any inborn error of amino acid metabolism that results in an accumulation of one or more amino acids in the blood or excess excretion in the urine, or both.

Apoptosis   When the secretory epithelial cells die and are reabsorbed.

Autocrine response   When a cell secretes a hormone/chemical that acts on itself.

Complementary feeding   The introduction of foods and drinks after six months of age. These foods are in addition to adequate intake of breastmilk.

Erythema   Redness of the skin.

Exclusive breastfeeding   Where the infant receives only breastmilk from its mother or expressed or donor breastmilk. No other liquids or solids, except vitamins or medicines, are given.

Fissure   Crack or tear in the skin.

Galactopoesis   Maintenance of lactation once it has been established.

Glucogenesis   Breakdown of glycogen to form gluscose.

Hepatosplenomegaly   Enlargement of the liver and spleen.

Ketogenesis   Production of ketone bodies resulting from fatty acid breakdown.

Lactocyte   Milk-producing cell.

Lactogenesis   The initiation of milk production.

Let-down reflex   Involuntary reflex that causes milk ejection.

Lipolysis   The breakdown of fat into glycerol and fatty acids as a source of energy.

Myoepethelial cells   Smooth muscle around the alveoli that contracts to stimulate milk ejection.

Neuroendocrine resonse   Interaction between nervous system and endocrine system.

Oedema   Accumulation of extracellular fluid.

Oxytocin   Pituitary hormone that stimulates contraction of the myoepethelial cells around the alveoli to stimulate milk ejection.

Prolactin   Pituitary hormone that stimulates and maintains milk production.

Prolactin inhibiting factor   Hypothalamic substance that inhibits the synthesis and release of prolactin.

Sucking   Action of drawing the breast into the mouth to create a vacuum.

Suckling   Combined characteristics of feeding at the breast, including sucking, swallowing and breathing.

Supplementary feeding   Feeds given to a baby under six months old to supplement its intake of breastmilk, where this is insufficient.

Tongue-tie   Abnormal shortness or thickness of the frenulum that results in restricted tongue movement or anchorage to the base of the mouth.

References

Adamson, J. (2004) Implementing Informed Choice on Infant Feeding, *British Journal of Midwifery*, 12(9): 586–90.

Alban-Davies, H., Clark, J., Dalton, K. *et al.* (1989) Insulin Requirements of Diabetic Women who Breastfeed, *British Medical Journal*, 298: 1357–8.

Albright, L. (2003) Sore Nipples in Breastfeeding Mothers: Causes and Treatment, *International Journal of Pharaceutical Compounding*, 7(6): 426–33.

Al-Nassaj, H., Al-Ward, N. and Al-Awqati, N. (2004) Knowledge, Attitudes and Sources of Information on Breastfeeding among Medical Professionals in Baghdad, *Eastern Mediterranean Health Journal*, 10(6): 871–8.

Alyoysius, A. and Lozano, S. (2007) Provision of Nipple Shields to Preterm Infants on a Neonatal Unit: A Survey of Current Practice, *MIDIRS Midwifery Digest*, 17(3): 419–22.

Amir, L. (2002) Does Maternal Smoking have a Negative Physiological Effect on Breastfeeding? The Epidemiological Evidence, *Birth*, 29(2): 112–23.

Anderson, J., Held, N. and Wright, K. (2004) Raynaud's Phenomenon of the Nipple: A Treatable Cause of Nipple Pain, *Pediatrics*, 113(4): 360–4.

Armstrong, J. and Reilly, J. (2002) Breastfeeding and Lowering the Risk of Childhood Obesity, *The Lancet*, 359(9322): 2003–4.

Ball, H. (2002) Reasons to Bed-share: Why Parents Sleep with their Infants, *Journal of Reproductive and Infant Psychology*, 20(4): 207–21.

Ball, H. (2003) Breastfeeding, Bed-sharing, and Infant Sleep, *Birth*, 30(3): 181–8.

Ball, H. (2009) Bed-sharing and Co-sleeping, *Perspective NCT*, (5): 10–2.

Ball, H., Ward-Platt, M., Heslop, E. *et al.* (2006) Randomised Trial of Infant Sleep Location on the Postnatal Ward, *Archive of Disease in Childhood*, 91(12): 1005–10.

Battersby, S. (2002) Midwives' Embodied Knowledge of Breastfeeding, *MIDIRS Midwifery Digest*, 12(4): 523–6.

Baxter, J. (2006) Women's Experience of Infant Feeding Following Birth by Caesarean Section, *British Journal of Midwifery*, 14(5): 290–5.

Bergman, N. (2008) Breastfeeding and Perinatal Neuroscience, in C.W. Genna (ed.) *Supporting Suckling Skills in Breastfeeding Infants* (pp. 43–56), London: Jones and Bartlett.

Bergman, N., Linley, L. and Faweus, S. (2004) Randomised Control Trial of Skin-to-Skin Contact from Birth Versus Conventional Incubator for Physiological Stabilisation in 1200–2199 Gram Newborns, *Acta Paediatrica*, 93(6): 779–85.

Berry, C., Thomas, E., Piper, K. *et al.* (2007) The Histology and Cytology of the Human Mammary Gland and Breastmilk, in T. Hale and P. Hartman (eds) *Textbook of Human Lactation* (pp. 35–47). Amarillo, TX: Hale Publishing.

BFN (Breastfeeding Network) (2002) *Assessing the Evidence: Cracked Nipples and Wound Healing*, Paisley: BFN.

BFN (Breastfeeding Network) (2008) *Differential Diagnosis of Nipple Pain*. Available online at www.breastfeedingnetwork.org.uk/pdfs/differenetialdiagnosisofnipplepain-June%2008.pdf (accessed 28 October 2008).

BFN (Breastfeeding Network) (2009a) *Expressing and Storing Breast Milk*. Available online at www.breastfeedingnetwork.org.uk/pdfs/BFNExpressing&Storing.pdf (accessed 7 March 2010).

BFN (Breastfeeding Network) (2009b) *Mastitis and Breastfeeding*, Paisley: BFN.

BFN (Breastfeeding Network) (2009c) *Thrush and Breastfeeding*, Paisley: BFN.

Bishop, H., Cousins, W., Casson, K. *et al.* (2008) Culture and Caregivers: Factors Influencing Breastfeeding among Mothers in West Belfast, Northern Ireland, *Child Care in Practice*, 14(2): 165–79.

Blair, P., Sidebotham, P., Evason-Coombe, C. *et al.* (2009) Hazardos Cosleeping Environments and Risk Factors Amenable to Change: Case-control Study of SIDS in South West England, *British Medical Journal*, 339: b3666. Available online at www.bmj.com/content/339/bmj.b3666.full (accessed 7 April 2100).

Bolling, K., Grant, C., Hamlyn, B. *et al.* (2007) *Infant Feeding Survey 2005*, London: The Information Centre.

Both, D. and Frischknect, K. (2008) *Breastfeeding: An Illustrated Guide to Diagnosis and Treatment*, Edinburgh: Mosby Elsevier.

Boud, D., Keogh, R. and Walker, D. (eds) (1985) *Reflection: Turning Experience into Learning*, London: Kogan Page.

Briton, C., McCormick, E., Renfrew, M. *et al.* (2007) Support for Breastfeeding Mothers (Review), *Cochrane Database of Systematic Reviews*, 1: Art. No. CD001141. DOI: 10.1002/14561858. CD001141.pub3.

Britten, J. and Broadfoot, M. (2002) Breastfeeding Support in Scotland, *British Journal of Midwifery*, 10(5): 292–6.

Britten, J., Hoddinott, P. and McInnes, R. (2006) Breastfeeding Peer Support: Health Service Programmes in Scotland, *British Journal of Midwifery*, 14(1): 12–8.

Broadfoot, M., Britten, J., Tappin, D. *et al.* (2005a) The Baby Friendly Hospital Initiative and Breastfeeding Rates in Scotland, *Archives of Disease in Childhood: Fetal and Neonatal Edition*, 90: 114–6.

Broadfoot, M., Britten, J., Tappin, D. *et al.* (2005b) The Baby Friendly Hospital Initiative and Breastfeeding Rates in Scotland, *Archives of Disease in Childhood: Fetal and Neonatal Edition*, 90: 114–16).

Buckley, K. (2009) A Double-Edged Sword: Lactation Consultants' Perceptions of the Impact of Breast Pumps on the Practice of Breastfeeding, *Journal of Perinatal Education*, 18(2): 13–22.

Cairney, P. and Alder, E. (2001) A Survey of Information Given by Health Professionals, about Bottle Feeding, to First Time Mothers in a Scottish Population, *Health Bulletin*, 59(2): 97–101.

Caldwell, K., Turner-Maffei, C., Blair, A. *et al.* (2004) Pain Reduction and Treatment of Sore Nipples in Nursing Mothers, *Journal of Perinatal Education*, 13(1): 29–35.

Cantrill, R., Creedy, D. and Cooke, M. (2003) How Midwives Learn About Breastfeeding, *Australian Midwifery Journal*, 16(2): 11–6.

Carper, B.A. (1978) Fundamental Patterns of Knowing in Nursing, *Advances in Nursing Science*, 1(1): 13–23.

Chertok, I. (2009) Reexamination of Ultra-thin Nipple Shield Use, Infant Growth and Maternal Satisfaction, *Journal of Clinical Nursing*, 18(21): 2049–55.

Chertok, I., Raz, I., Shoham, I. *et al.* (2009) Effects of Early Breastfeeding on Neonatal Glucose Levels of Term Infants Born to Women with Gestational Diabetes, *Journal of Human Nutrition and Dietetics*, 22(2): 166–9.

Colson, S. (2010) *Biological Nurturing: Laid Back Breastfeeding*. Available online at www. biologicalnurturing.com (accessed 6 August 2010).

Conde-Agudelo, A. and Belizan, J. (2009) Kangaroo Mother Care to Reduce Morbidity and Mortality in Low Birthweight Infants, *Cochrane Database of Systematic Reviews*, 2: Art. No.: CD002771. DOI:10:1002/14651858.CD002771.

Coppa, G., Bruni, S., Morelli, L. *et al.* (2004) The First Prebiotics in Humans: Human Milk Oligosaccharides, *Journal of Clinical Gastroenterology*, 38: 80–3.

Cox, D., Owens, R. and Hartmann, P. (1996) Blood and Milk Prolactin and the Rate of Milk Synthesis in Women, *Experimental Physiology*, 81: 1007–20.

Craig, J. (2002) How to Ask the Right Question, in J. Craig and R. Smyth (eds) *The Evidence-based Practice Manual for Nurses* (pp. 24–44), London: Churchill Livingstone.

Cregan, M., Mitoulas, L. and Hartmann, P. (2002) Milk Prolactin, Feed Volume and Duration between Feeds in Women Breastfeeding their Full-term Infants over a 24h Period, *Experimental Physiology*, 87(2): 207–14. Available online at http://ep.physoc.org/cgi/reprint/87/2/207.pdf (accessed 9 April 2011).

Czank, C., Henderson, J., Kent, J. *et al.* (2007) Hormonal Control of the Lactation Cycle, in T. Hale and P. Hartmann (eds) *Textbook of Human Lactation* (pp. 89–112), Amarillo, TX: Hale Publishing.

Czank, C., Mitoulas, L.R. and Hartmann, P. (2007) Human Milk Composition: Fat, in T. Hale and P. Hartmann (eds) *Textbook of Human Lactation* (p. 49–68). Amarillo, TX: Hale Publishing.

Dewey, K., Nommsen-Rivers, L. and Heinig, J. (2005) Risk Factors for Suboptimal Infant Breastfeeding Behaviour, Delayed Onset of Lactogenesis, and Excessive Neonatal Weight Loss, *Pediatrics*, 112: 607–19.

DH (Department of Health) (2000) *Hepatitis B Testing in Pregnancy: Information for Midwives*, London: DH.

DH (Department of Health) (2003a) *Essence of Care: Benchmarks for Communication between Patients, Carers and Healthcare Personnel*, London: DH.

DH (Department of Health) (2003b) *Infant Feeding Recommendations*. Available online at www.breastfeeding.nhs.uk/en/docs/FINAL_QA.pdf (accessed 15 May 2010).

DH (Department of Health) (2004a) *Breastfeeding Awareness Week Survey*, London: DH.

DH (Department of Health) (2004b) *Good Practice and Innovation in Breastfeeding*, London: DH.

DH (Department of Health) (2004c) *HIV and Infant Feeding: Guidance from the UK Chief Medical Officer's Expert Advisory Group*, London: DH.

DH (Department of Health) (2006) *How Much is Too Much? Pregnancy and Alcohol*, London: DH.

DH (Department of Health) (2007a) *Bottle Feeding*. Available online at www.dh.gov.uk/prod_consum_dh/groups/dh_digitalassets/documents/digitalasset/dh_084165.pdf (accessed 27 May 2010).

DH (Department of Health) (2007b) *Hepatitis B: How to Protect Your Baby*, London: DH.

DH (Department of Health) (2008) *Weaning: Starting Solid Food*. Available online at www.dh.gov.uk/prod_consum_dh/groups/dh_digitalassets/documents/digitalasset/dh_084164.pdf (accessed 23 May 2010).

DH (Department of Health) (2009a) *The Pregnancy Book 2009*, London DH.

DH (Department of Health) (2009b) *Taste for Life*. Available online at www.nhs.uk/start4life/pages/taste-for-life.aspx (accessed 25 August 2010).

DH (Department of Health) (2009c) *Using the New UK-World Health Organization 0–4 Years Growth Charts*, London COI.

DH (Department of Health) (2010a) *Breastfeeding and Introducing Solid Foods: Consumer Insight Summary*, London: DH.

DH (Department of Health) (2010b) *Review of the Controls on Infant Formula and Follow-on Infant Formula*. Available online at www.dh.gov.uk (accessed 18 July 2010).

DH (Department of Health) (2010c) *Start4life: A Good Start to a Healthier Life*, London: COI for Department of Health.

Dickens, V. (2008) Learning on the Job: Influences on the Initiation and Duration of Breastfeeding, *MIDIRS Midwifery Digest*, 18(2): 243–7.

DiGirolamo, A., Grummer-Strawn, L. and Fein, S. (2008) Effect of Maternity Care Practices on Breastfeeding, *Pediatrics*, 1: 22, 43–9.

Dodgson, J. and Tarrant, M. (2007) Outcomes of a Breastfeeding Educational Intervention for Baccalaureate Nursing Students, *Nurse Education Today*, 27(8): 856–67.

Dorea, J. (2007) Maternal Smoking and Infant Feeding: Breastfeeding is Better and Safer, *Maternal and Child Health*, 11: 287–91.

Dryden, C., Young, D., Hepburn, M. *et al.* (2009) Maternal Methadone Use in Pregnancy: Factors Associated with the Development of Neonatal Abstinence Syndrome and Implications for Healthcare Resources, *British Journal of Obstetrics and Gynaecology*, 116: 665–71.

Dungy, C., McInnes, R., Tappin, D. *et al.* (2008) Infant Feeding Attitudes and Knowledge among Socioeconomically Disadvantaged Women in Glasgow, *Maternal and Child Health*, 12: 313–22.

Dykes, F. (2003) Protecting, Promoting and Supporting Breastfeeding, *British Journal of Midwifery*, 11(10): 24–48.

Dykes, F. (2005) Government Funded Breastfeeding Support Projects: Implications for Practice, *Maternal and Child Nutrition*, 1(2): 21–31.

Dyson, L., Renfrew, M., McFadden, A. *et al.* (2006) *Promotion of Initiation and Duration of Breastfeeding: Evidence into Practice Briefing*, London: NICE.

Fawcett, J., Watson, J., Neuman, B. *et al.* (2001) On Nursing Theories and Evidence, *Journal of Nursing Scholarship*, Second quarter: 115–9.

Finigan, V. (2009) 'It's on the Tip of My Tongue': Evaluation of a New Frenulotomy Service in Northern England, *MIDIRS Midwifery Digest*, 19(3): 395–400.

Fisher, D. (1998) *Social Drugs and Breastfeeding*. Available online at www.health-e-learning.com (accessed 6 August 2010).

Flint, A., New, K. and Davies, M. (2007) Cup Feeding Versus Other Forms of Supplemental Enteral Feeding for Newborn Infants Unable to Fully Breastfeed, *Cochrane Database of Systematic Reveiws*, 2: Art. No. CD005092. DOI: 10.1002/14651858.CD005092.pub2.

Freed, G., Clark, S., Cefalo, R. *et al.* (1995) Breastfeeding Education of Obstetrics- Gynaecology Residents and Practitioners, *American Journal of Obstetrics and Gynaecology*, 173(5): 1607–13.

Freed, G., Clark, S., Harris, B. *et al.* (1996) Methods and Outcomes of Breastfeeding Instruction for Nursing Students, *Journal of Human Lactation*, 12: 105–10.

FSA (Food Standards Agency) (2010a) *FSA Powdered Infant Formula Research*. Available online at www.food.gov.uk (accessed 28 May 2010).

FSA (Food Standards Agency) (2010b) *Healthy Diet*. Available online at www.eatwell.gov.uk/healthydiet/nutritionessentials/milkanddairy (accessed 26 May 2010).

FSID (Foundation for the Study of Infant Deaths) (2009) *Dummy Information*. Available online at http://fsid.org.uk/Page.aspx?pid=416 (accessed 27 June 2010).

Gatti, L. (2008) Maternal Perceptions of Insufficient Milk Supply in Breastfeeding, *Journal of Nursing Scholarship*, 40(4): 355–63.

Geddes, D. (2007a) Gross Anatomy of the Lactating Breast, in T. Hale and P. Hartmann (eds) *Textbook of Human Lactation* (pp. 19–34), Amarillo TX: Hale Publishing.

Geddes, D. (2007b) Inside the Lactating Breast: The Latest Anatomy Research, *Journal of Midwifery and Women's Health*, 52(6): 556–63.

Geddes, D., Langton, D. and Gallow, I. (2008) Frenulotomy for Breastfeeding Infants with Ankyloglossia: Effect on Milk Removal and Sucking Mechanism as Imaged by Ultrasound, *Pediatrics*, 122(1): 188–94.

Genna, C.W. (2008) *Supporting Sucking Skills in Breastfeeding*, London: Jones and Bartlett Publishers.

Gibbs, G. (1998) *Learning by Doing: A Guide to Teaching and Learning Methods*, London: Further Education Unit.

Giglia, R. and Binns, C. (2008) Alcohol, Pregnancy and Breastfeeding: A Comparison of the 1995 and 2001 National Health Surveys, *Breastfeeding Review*, 16(1): 17–24.

Giglia, R., Binns, C., and Alfonso, H. (2006) Maternal Cigarette Smoking and Breastfeeding Duration, *Acta Paediatrica*, 95: 1370–4.

Gilks, J., Gould, D. and Price, E. (2008) Decontaminating Breast Pump Collection Kits for Use on a Neonatal Unit, *MIDIRS Midwifery Digest*, 18(2): 256–9.

Gray, J. (2001) *Evidence Based Health Care* (2nd edn), London: Churchill Livingstone.

Grummer-Strawn, L. and Mei, Z. (2004) Does Breastfeeding Protect against Pediatric Overweight? Analysis of Longitudinal Data from the Centers for Disease Control and Prevention Pediatric Nutrition Surveillance System, *Pediatrics*, 113: 81–6.

Hake-Brooks, S. and Anderson, G. (2008) Kangaroo Care and Breastfeeding of Mother-Preterm Infant Dyads 0–18 Months: A Randomised Controlled Trial, *Neonatal Network*, 27: 151–9.

Hale, T. (2008) *Medications and Mothers Milk*, Amarillo, TX: Pharmasoft Medical Publishing.

Hale, T. and Hartmann, P. (eds) (2007) *Textbook of Human Lactation*, Amarillo, TX: Hale Publishing.

Hale, T., Kristensen, J. and Ilett, K. (2007) The Transfer of Medications into Human Milk, in T. Hale and P. Hartmann (eds) *Textbook of Human Lactation* (pp. 465–77), Amarillo, TX: Hale Publishing.

Hall-Moran, V., Dykes, F., Edwards, J. *et al.* (2004) An Evaluation of the Breastfeeding Support Skills of Midwives and Voluntary Breastfeeding Supporters Using the Breastfeeding Support Skill Tool (Besst), *Maternal and Child Nutrition*, 1: 241–9.

Hargreaves, K. and Harris, A. (2009) Nipple Confusion in Neonates, *British Journal of Midwifery*, 17(2): 97–103.

Hartmann, P. and Cregan, M. (2001) Lactogenesis and the Effects of Insulin-Dependent Diabetes Mellitus and Prematurity, *Journal of Nutrition*, 131: 3016–20.

Hartmann, P. and Ramsay, D. (2006) Mammary Anatomy and Physiology, in E. Jones and C. King (eds) *Feeding and Nutrition in the Preterm Infant*, London: Elsevier.

Health Promotion Agency (2004) *Peer Support as an Intervention to Increase the Incidence and Duration of Breastfeeding in Northern Ireland: What is the Evidence?* Belfast: Health Promotion Agency.

Health Protection Agency (2006) *Pregnancy and Tuberculosis*, London: HPA.

Health Scotland (2009) *Breastfeeding and Returning to Work*, Glasgow: Health Scotland.

Health Scotland (2010) *Fun First Foods: Briefing Paper for Professionals*. Available online at www.healthscotland.com/resources/publications (accessed 6 November 2010).

Heath, H. (1998) Reflection and Patterns of Knowing in Nursing, *Journal of Advanced Nursing*, 27: 1054–9.

Hellings, P. and Howe, C. (2004) Breastfeeding Knowledge and Practice of Pediatric Nurse Practitioners, *Journal of Pediatric Health Care*, 18(1): 8–14.

Hemingway, P. (2009) *What is a Systematic Review*. What is . . . ? Series. Available online at www.whatisseries.co.uk (accessed 5 September 2010).

Henderson, G., McGuire, A. and McGuire, W. (2007) Formula Milk Versus Maternal Breastmilk for Feeding Preterm or Low Weight Infants, *Cochrane Database of Systematic Reveiws*, 4: Art. No. CD002971. DOI:10.1002/14651858. CD002971.pub2.

Henderson, J., Hartmann, P. and Newham, J. (2008) Effects of Preterm Birth and Antenatal Corticosteroid Treatment on Lactogenesis II in Women, *Pediatrics*, 121, 92–100.

Hepatitis B Foundation (2007) *Hepatitis B Guidelines for Pregnant Women*. Available at www.hepb.org (accessed 25 July 2010).

Hepatitis B Foundation (2009) *Breastfeeding*. Available online at www.hepb.org (accessed 25 July 2010).

Hewitt, H. (2008) Peer Influence. *MIDIRS Midwifery Digest*, 18(2): 260–2.

Hilton, S. (2008) Milk Production During Pregnancy and Beyond, *British Journal of Midwifery*, 16(8): 544–8.

Hogan, M., Westcott, C. and Griffiths, M. (2005) Randomised Control Trial of Divsion of Tongue-Tie in Infants with Feeding Problems, *Journal of Paediatrics and Child Health*, 41(5–6): 246–50.

Horvath, T., Madi, B., Iuppa, I. *et al.* (2009) Interventions for Preventing Late Postnatal Mother-to-Child Transmission of HIV, *Cochrane Database of Systematic Reviews*, 1: Art. No.: CD006734. DOI: 10.1002/14651858.CD006734.pub2.

Howard, C.R., Howard, F.M., Lanaphear, B. *et al.* (2003) Randomised Clinical Trial of Pacifier Use and Bottle Feeding or Cup Feeding and Their Effect on Breastfeeding, *Pediatrics*, 111(3): 511–18.

HSE (Health and Safety Executive) (2009) *A Guide for New and Expectant Mothers Who Work*. Available online at www.hse.gov.uk/pubns/indg373.pdf (accessed 6 August 2010).

HSE (Health and Safety Executive) (2010) *Legislation Affecting New and Expectant Mothers at Work*. Available online at www.hse.gov.uk/mothers/law.htm (accessed 10 August 2010).

Hunter, G., Baykal, T., Demir, F. *et al.* (2005) Breastfeeding Experiences in Inborn Errors of Metabolism Other Than Phenylketonuria, *Journal of Inherited Metabolic Disorders*, 28(4): 457–65.

Hurst, N.M. (2007) Recognising and Treating Delayed or Failed Lactogenesis II, *Journal of Midwifery & Women's Health*, 52(6): 588–94.

Ingram, J. (2006) Multiprofessional Training for Breastfeeding Management in Primary Care in the UK, *International Breastfeeding Journal*, 1(9). Available online at www.international breastfeedingjournal.com/content/pdf/1746-4358-1-10.pdf (accessed 25 July 2010).

Ip, S., Raman, G., Chew, P. *et al.* (2007) *Breastfeeding and Maternal Health Outcomes in Developed Countries: Evidence Report/Technology Assessment No. 153*, Agency for Healthcare Research and Quality. Available online at www.ahrq.gov/downloads/pub/evidence/pdf/brfout/brfout.pdf (accessed 24 May 2010).

Iyer, N., Srinivasan, R., Evans, K. *et al.* (2008) Impact of Early Weighing Policy on Neonatal Hypernatraemic Dehydration and Breastfeeding, *Archives of Childhood Disease*, 93(4): 297–9.

Jackson, A. (2007) Breastfeeding Education and Professional Development in the North Trent Neonatal Network, *MIDIRS Midwifery Digest*, 17(1): 90–3.

Jackson, W. (2004) Breastfeeding and Type 1 Diabetes Mellitus, *British Journal of Midwifery*, 12(3): 158–65.

Jambert-Gray, R., Lucas, K. and Hall, V. (2009) Methadone-Treated Mothers: Pregnancy and Breastfeeding, *British Journal of Midwifery*, 17(10): 654–7.

Januszewski, A. (2001) *Educational Technology: The Development of a Concept*, USA: Libraries Unlimited Inc.

Johns, C. (1995) Framing Learning through Reflection within Carper's Fundamental Ways of Knowing in Nursing, *Journal of Advanced Nursing*, 22: 226–34.

Johnston, C., Filion, F. and Campbell-Yeo, M. (2008) Kangaroo Mother Care Diminishes Pain from Heel Lance in Very Preterm Infants: A Cross-over Trial, *MIDIRS Midwifery Digest*, 18(4): 574–5.

Jonas, W., Nissen, E., Ransjo-Arvidson, A. *et al.* (2008) Short and Long Term Decrease of Blood Pressure in Women During Breastfeeding, *Breastfeed Medicine*, 3: 103–9.

Jones, E. and Spencer, S. (2008) Optimising the Provision of Human Milk in Preterm Infants, *MIDIRS Midwifery Digest*, 18(1): 118–21.

Jones, W. (2008) Giving Advice on Breastfeeding, *The Pharmaceutical Journal*, 280: 723–6.

Jones, W. (2009a) *Creams and Ointments Applied to the Skin of Breastfeeding Mothers.* Available online at www.breastfeedingnetwork.org.uk/pdfs/Creams_and_Ointments_and_Breastfeeding_March_2009.pdf (accessed 25 July 2010).

Jones, W. (2009b) *Differential Diagnosis of Nipple Pain*, Paisley: BFN.

Jones, W. (2009c) *Increasing Milk Supply: Use of Galactagogues.* Available online at www.breastfeedingnetwork.org.uk (accessed 30 September 2010).

Jones, W. (2009d) *Smoking and Breastfeeding.* Available online at www.breastfeedingnetwork.org.uk/pdfs/Smoking_and_Breastfeeding_March_2009.pdf (accessed 4 October 2010).

Kanufre, V., Starling, A., Leao, E. et al. (2007) Breastfeeding and the Treatment of Children with Phenylketonuria, *Journal of Pediatrics*, 83(5): 447–52.

Kent, J. (2007) How Breastfeeding Works, *Journal of Midwifery & Women's Health*, 52(6): 564–70.

Kent, J., Mitoulas, L., Cregan, M. et al. (2006) Volume and Frequency of Breastfeedings and Fat Content of Breastmilk Throughout the Day, *Pediatrics*, 117(3): 387–95.

Kent, J., Mitoulas, L., Cregan, M. et al. (2008) Importance of Vacuum for Breastmilk Expression, *Breastfeed Medicine*, 3: 11–9.

Khan, F., Green, F., Forsyth, J. et al. (2009) The Beneficial Effects of Breastfeeding on Microvascular Function in 11 to 14 Year Old Children, *Vascular Medicine*, 14: 137–42.

Knight, C., Peaker, M. and Wilde, C. (1998) Local Control of Mammary Development and Function, *Reviews of Reproduction*, 3: 104–12.

Kramer, M., Aboud, F. and Mironova, E. (2008) Breastfeeding and Child Cognitive Development: New Evidence from a Large Randomised Trial, *Archives of General Psychiatry*, 65: 578–84.

Kronborg, H., Vaeth, M., Olsen, O. et al. (2007) Health Visitors and Breastfeeding Support: Influence of Knowledge and Self-Efficacy, *European Journal of Public Health*, 18(3): 283–8.

La Leche League International (2006) *Breastfeeding During Pregnancy.* Available online at www.llli.org/FAQ/bfpregnant.html (accessed 7 March 2010).

La Leche League International (2009) *What Are the LLLI Guidelines for Storing My Pumped Milk?* Available online at www.llli.org/FAQ/milkstorage.html (accessed 7 March 2010).

Ladhani, S., Srinivasan, L., Buchanan, C. et al. (2004) Presentation of Vitamin D Deficiency, *Archives of Disease in Childhood*, 89: 781–4.

Lawrence, R. and Lawrence, R. (2005) *Breastfeeding: A Guide for the Medical Profession* (6th edn), St Louis, MO: Mosby.

Lee-Dennis, C., Allen, K., McCormick, F. et al. (2009) Interventions for Treating Painful Nipples among Breastfeeding Women, *Cochrane Database of Systematic Reveiws*, 4: Art. No. CD007366. DOI:10:1002/14651858.CD007366.

Leon-Cava, N., Lutter, C., Ross, J. et al. (2002) *The Benefits of Breastfeeding: A Summary of the Evidence*, Washington DC: PAHO.

Levene, M., Tudehope, D. and Sinha, S. (2008) *Essential Neonatal Medicine* (4th edn), London: Blackwell.

Lewallen, L.P., Dick, M., Flowers, J. et al. (2006) Breastfeeding Support and Early Cessation, *Journal of Obstetrics, Gynaecology and Neonatal Nursing*, 35(2): 166–72.

Li, R., Fein, S., Chen, J. et al. (2008) Why Mothers Stop Breastfeeding: Mothers' Self-reported Reasons for Stopping During the First Year, *Pediatrics*, 122(Supplement 2): 569–76.

Livingstone, V. (1996) Too Much of a Good Thing: Maternal and Infant Hyperlactation Syndromes, *Canadian Family Physician*, 42: 89–99.

Livingstone, V., Willis, C., Abdel-Wareth, L. et al. (2000) Neonatal Hypernatraemic Dehydration, *Canadian Medical Association Journal*, 162(5): 647–52.

Lubbers, C.A. (1990) Communication Skills for Continuing Education in Nursing, *Journal of Continuing Education in Nursing*, 21(3): 109–12.

Liu, B., Beral, V. and Balkwall, A. (2008) Childbearing, Breastfeeding, Other Reproductive Factors and the Subsequent Risk of Hospitalization for Gallbladder Disease, *International Journal of Epidemiology*, 1–7. Available online at http://ije.oxfordjournals.org/content/early/2008/09/04/ije.dyn174.short (accessed 7 April 2010).

McAfee, G. (2007) Drugs of Abuse and Breastfeeding, in T. Hale and P. Hartmann (eds) *Textbook of Human Lactation* (pp. 575–609), Amarillo, TX: Hale Publishing.

McCrory, F. and Richens, Y. (2007) Pregnancy, Parenting and Substance Misuse, in Y. Richens (ed.) *Challenges for Midwives Volume II* (pp. 201–13), London: Quay Books.

McFadden, A., Renfrew, M.J., Wallace, L. *et al.* (2007) Does Breastfeeding Really Matter? A National Multidisciplinary Breastfeeding Knowledge and Skills Assessment, *MIDIRS Midwifery Digest*, 17(1): 85–8.

McGrath, J. and Braescu, A. (2004) State of the Science Feeding Readiness in the Preterm Infant, *Journal of Perinatal and Neonatal Nursing*, Oct–Dec: 353–70.

McInnes, R. and Chambers, J. (2006) *Breastfeeding in Neonatal Units: A Review of Breastfeeding Publications between 1990–2005*, Edinburgh: NHS Health Scotland/Scottish Executive.

McInnes, R. and Chambers, J. (2008a) Infants Admitted to Neonatal Units – Interventions to Improve Breastfeeding Outcomes: A Systematic Review 1990–2007, *Maternal and Child Health*, 4: 235–63.

McInnes, R. and Chambers, J. (2008b) Supporting Breastfeeding Mothers: Qualitative Synthesis, *Journal of Advanced Nursing*, 62(4): 407–27.

Mangesi, L. and Dowswell, T. (2010) Treatments for Breast Engorgement During Lactation, *Cochrane Database of Systematic Reveiws*, 9: Art. No. CD006946. DOI:10.1002/14651858. CD006946.pub2.

Mannella, J., Yourshaw, L. and Morgan, L. (2007) Breastfeeding and Smoking: Short-term Effects on Infant Feeding and Sleep, *Pediatrics*, 120(3): 497–502.

Marasco, L. and Marmet, C. (2000) Polycystic Ovary Syndrome: A Connection to Insufficient Milk Supply, *Journal of Human Lactation*, 16(2): 143–8.

Martyn, T. (2003) Infant Feeding, *Midwives*, 6(5): 215.

Matthiesen, A.S., Ransjo-Ardvison, A.B., Nissen, E. *et al.* (2001) Postpartum Maternal Oxytocin Release by Newborns: Effects of Infant Hand Massage and Sucking, *Birth*, 28(1): 20–1.

Menella, J. and Pepino, M. (2008) Biphasic Effects of Moderate Drinking on Prolactin During Lactation, *Alcoholism: Clinical and Experimental Research*, 32(11): 1899–908.

Merten, S., Dratva, J. and Ackermann-Liebrich, U. (2005) Do Baby Friendly Hospitals Influence Breastfeeding Duration on a National Level? *Pediatrics*, 116(5): 702–8.

Moberg, K. (2003) *The Oxytocin Factor: Tapping the Hormone of Calm, Loving and Healing*, Cambridge MA: Da Capo Press.

Moore, E., Anderson, G. and Bergman, N. (2009) Early Skin-to-skin Contact for Mothers and their Healthy Newborn Infants, *Cochrane Database of Systematic Reveiws*, 3: Art. No. CD003519. DOI: 10.1002/14651858.CD0035.pub2.

Moser, K., Whittle, C. and Hicks, C. (2003) Social Inequalities in Low Birth Weight in England and Wales: Trends and Implications for Future Population Health, *Journal of Epidemiology and Community Health*, 57: 687–91.

Muirhead, P., Butcher, G., Rankin, J. *et al.* (2006) The Effect of a Programme of Organised and Supervised Peer Support on the Initiation and Duration of Breastfeeding: A Randomised Controlled Trial, *British Journal of General Practice*, 56(524): 191–7.

National Statistics (2005) *National Statistics Socio-economic Classification: Origins, Development and Use*, Basingstoke: Palgrave Macmillan.

Neifert, M., Lawrence, R. and Seacat, J. (1995) Nipple Confusion: Towards a Formal Definition, *Journal of Pediatrics*, 126(6): 125–9.

NHS Choices (2009) *Is It Safe to Drink Alcohol While Breastfeeding?* Available online at www.nhs.uk (accessed 7 July 2010).

NHS Information Centre (2010) *Statistics on Obesity, Physical Activity and Diet: England, 2010*, London: The Health and Social Care Information Centre.

NICE (2004) The Epilepsies: The Diagnosis and Management of the Epilepsies in Adults and Children in Primary and Secondary Care, London: NICE.

NICE (2005) *Division of Ankyloglossia (Tongue-tie) for Breastfeeding*, Ipg149, London: NICE.

NICE (2006a) *Routine Postnatal Care of Women and Their Babies*, London: NICE.

NICE (2006b) *Routine Postnatal Care of Women and Their Babies: Costing Report*, London: NICE.

NICE (2008a) *Antenatal Care: Routine Care for Healthy Pregnant Women*, London: NICE.

NICE (2008b) *Diabetes in Pregnancy: Management of Diabetes and its Complications from Pre-conception to the Postnatal Period*, London: NICE.

NICE (2008c) *Maternal and Child Nutrition: Improving the Nutrition of Pregnant and Breastfeeding Mothers and Children in Low-income Households*, London: NICE.

NICE (2010) *Donor Breast Milk Banks: Nice Clinical Guideline 93*, London: NICE.

Nickell, W.B. and Skelton, J. (2005) Breast Fat and Fallicies, *Journal of Human Lactation*, 21(2): 126–30.

Nissen, E., Uvnas-Moberg, K., Svensson, K. *et al.* (1996) Different Patterns of Oxytocin, Prolactin but not Cortisil Release during Breastfeeding in Women Delivered by Caesarean Section or by the Vaginal Route, *Early Human Development*, 45: 103–18.

NMC (Nursing and Midwifery Council) (2007a) *Essential Skills Clusters (ESCs) for Pre-registration Midwifery Education: Nursing and Midwifery Council Circular 23/2007*, London: NMC.

NMC (Nursing and Midwifery Council) (2008) *The Code: Standards of Conduct, Performance and Ethics for Nurses and Midwives*, London: NMC.

NMC (Nursing and Midwifery Council) (2009) *Standards for Pre-registration Midwifery Education*, London: NMC.

Nommsen-Rivers, L. (2003) Cosmetic Breast Surgery: Is Breastfeeding at Risk? *Journal of Human Lactation*, 19(7): 7–8.

Nommsen-Rivers, L., Heinig, M., Cohen, R. *et al.* (2008) Newborn Wet and Soiled Diaper Counts and Timing of Onset of Lactation as Indicators of Breastfeeding Inadequacy, *Journal of Human Lactation*, 24: 27–33.

Noon, M. (2010) Lactational Mastitis: Recognition and Breastfeeding Support, *British Journal of Midwifery*, 18(8): 503–8.

O'Brien, M., Buikstra, E., Fallon, T. *et al.* (2009) Strategies for Success: A Tool Box of Coping Strategies Used by Breastfeeding Women, *Journal of Clinical Nursing*, 18: 1574–82.

Osborn, D. and Sinn, J. (2006) Soya Formula for Prevention of Allergy and Food Intolerance in Infants, *Cochrane Database of Systematic Reviews*, 4: Art. No. CD003741. DOI: 10.1002/14651858.CD003741.pub4.

Osborn, D. and Sinn, J. (2007) Prebiotics in Infants for Prevention of Allergic Disease and Food Hypersensitivity, *Cochrane Database of Systematic Reviews*, 4: Art. No. CD006474. DOI: 10.1002/14651858.CD006474.pub2

Owen, C., Wincupp, P., Kaye, S. *et al.* (2008) Does Initial Breastfeeding Lead to Lower Blood Cholesterol in Adult Life? A Quantitative Review of the Evidence, *American Journal of Clinical Nutrition*, 88: 305–14.

Paley, J., Cheyne, H., Dalgleish, L. *et al.* (2007) Nursing's Ways of Knowing and Dual Process Theories of Cognition, *Journal of Advanced Nursing*, 60(6): 692–701.

Palmer, G. (2009) *The Politics of Breastfeeding* (3rd edn), London: Pinter and Martin.

Parahoo, K. (2006) *Nursing Research: Principles, Process and Issues* (2nd edn), Basingstoke: Wilkins.

Pikwer, M., Bergstrom, U., Nilsson, J. *et al.* (2008) Breastfeeding, But Not Oral Contraceptives, is Associated with a Reduced Risk of Rheumatoid Arthritis, *Annals of the Rheumatic Diseases*. Available online at http://ard.bmj.com/content/early/2008/05/13/ard.2007.084707.abstract (accessed 6 August 2010).

Pollard, M. (2010) Learning about Breastfeeding in a Baby Friendly Accredited Pre-registration Midwifery Programme, unpublished EdD thesis, University of Strathclyde.

Prime, D., Geddes, D. and Hartmann, P. (2007) Oxytocin: Milk Ejection and Maternal–Infant Well-being, in T. Hale and P. Hartmann (eds) *Textbook of Human Lactation* (pp. 141–55), Amarillo, TX: Hale Publishing.

Quigley, M., Henderson, G., Anthony, M. *et al.* (2007) Formula Milk Versus Donor Breast Milk for Feeding Preterm or Low Birth Weight Infants, *Cochrane Database of Systematic Reviews*, 4: Art. No. CD002971. DOI: 10.1002/14651858.CD002971.pub2.

Ramsay, D.T., Kent, J.C., Hartmann, R.A. *et al.* (2005) Anatomy of the Lactating Breast Redefined with Ultrasound Imaging, *Journal of Anatomy*, 206(6): 525–34.

Rapley, G. (2006) Baby-led Weaning: A Developmental Approach to the Introduction of Complementary Foods, in V. Hall-Moran and F. Dykes (eds) *Maternal and Infant Nutrition and Nurture: Controversies and Challenges* (pp. 275–98), London: Quay Books.

Rapley, G. (2008) *Baby-led Weaning*. Available online at www.rapleyweaning.com/assets/blw leaflet.pdf (accessed 9 March 2011).

Rasmussen, K. (2007) Maternal Obesity and the Outcome of Breastfeeding, in T. Hale and P. Hartmann (eds) *Textbook of Human Lactation* (pp. 387–402), Amarillo, TX: Hale Publishing.

Rasmussen, K. and Kjolhede, C. (2004) Pre-pregnant Overweight and Obesity Diminish the Prolactin Response to Suckling in the First Week Postpartum, *Pediatrics*, 113: 465–71.

RCM (Royal College of Midwifery) (2009) *Infant Feeding: A Resource for Health Care Professionals and Parents*, London: RCM Trust.

Remmington, S. and Remmington, T. (2009) Early Additional Food and Fluids for Healthy Breastfed Full-term Infants (Protocol), *Cochrane Database of Systematic Reveiws*, 2: Art. No. CD006462. DOI:10:1002/146518.CD006462.

Renfrew, M., Ansell, P. and MacLeod, K. (2003) Formula Feed Preparation: Helping Reduce the Risks: A Systematic Review, *Archives of Disease in Childhood*, 88(10): 855–8.

Renfrew, M., Dyson, L., McCormick, E. *et al.* (2009) Breastfeeding Promotion for Infants in Neonatal Units: A Systematic Review, *Child: Care, Health and Development*, 36(2): 165–78.

Renfrew, M., Dyson, L., Wallace, L. *et al.* (2005) *The Effectiveness of Public Health Interventions to Promote the Duration of Breastfeeding: Systematic Review*, London: NICE.

Renfrew, M., McLoughlin, M. and McFadden, A. (2008) Cleaning and Sterilisation of Infant Feeding Equipment: A Systematic Review, *Public Health Nutrition*, 11(11): 1188–99.

Renfrew, M., Woolridge, M. and McGill, H.R. (2000) *Enabling Women to Breastfeed: A Review of Practices which Promote or Inhibit Breastfeeding – with Evidence-based Guidance for Practice*, London: The Stationery Office.

Retallack, S., Simmer, K., Makrides, M. *et al.* (2008) Infant Weaning Practices in Adelaide: The Results of a Shopping Complex Survey, *Journal of Paediatrics and Child Health*, 30(1): 28–32.

Rocha, N.M., Martinez, M.E. and Jorge, S.M. (2002) Cup or Bottle for Premature Infants: Effects on Oxygen Saturation, Weight Gain, and Breastfeeding, *Journal of Human Lactation*, 18: 132–8.

Roller, C. (2005) Getting to Know Mothers' Experiences of Kangaroo Care, *Journal of Obstetrics, Gynaecology and Neonatal Nursing*, 34: 210–17.

Rowe-Murray, H. and Fisher, J. (2002) Baby Friendly Hospital Practices: Caesarean Section is a Persistent Barrier to Early Initiation of Breastfeeding, *Birth*, 29: 124–31.

Sackett, D., Rosenberg, W., Gray, J. *et al.* (1996) Evidence Based Medicine: What It Is and What It Isn't, *British Medical Journal*, 312: 71–2.

SACN (Scientific Advisory Committee on Nutrition) (2007a) *SMCN Response to the Infant Formula and Follow-on Formula Draft Regulations 2007: Position Statement by the Scientific Advisory Committee on Nutrition 2007*. Available online at www.sacn.gov.uk/pdfs/position_statement_2007_09_24.pdf (accessed 9 April 2011).

SACN (Scientific Advisory Committee on Nutrition) (2007b) *Update on Vitamin D: Position Statement by the Scientific Advisory Committee on Nutrition 2007*, London: The Stationery Office.

SACN (Scientific Advisory Committee on Nutrition) (2008a) Consideration of the Place of 'Good Night' Milk Products in the Diet of Infants Aged 6 Months. Available online at www.sacn.gov.uk/pdfs/final_sacn_statement-on_good_night_milks.pdf (accessed 25 May 2010).

SACN (Scientific Advisory Committee on Nutrition) (2008b) *Infant Feeding Survey 2005: A Commentary on Infant Feeding Practices in the UK*, London: The Stationery Office.

Schaal, B., Doucet, S., Sagot, P. *et al.* (2005) Human Breast Areolae as Scent Organs: Morphological Data and Possible Involvement in Maternal–Neonatal Condition, *Developmental Psychobiology*, 48: 100=10.

Schön, D. (1983) *The Reflective Practitioner*, New York: Basic Books.

Breastfed Infants From Low Income Families, *Journal of Human Lactation*, 25: 11–17.

Scottish Government (2002) *Hepatitis C: Essential Information for Professionals*. Available at www.scotland.gov.uk/Publications/2002/07/15074/8614 (accessed 9 April 2011).

Sherburne-Hawkins, S., Cole, T. and Law, C. (2008) An Ecological Systems Approach to Examining Risk Factors for Early Childhood Overweight: Findings from the UK Millenium Cohort Study, *Journal of Epidemiology Community Health*, 63(2): 147–55. Available online at http://eprints.ucl.ac.uk/14503/1/14503.pdf (accessed 9 April 2011).

Sheriff, N., Hall, V. and Pickin, M. (2009) Fathers' Perspectives on Breastfeeding: Ideas for Intervention, *British Journal of Midwifery*, 17(4): 223–7.

SIGN (Scottish Intercollegiate Guidelines Network) (2003) *Diagnosis and Management of Epilepsy in Adults: Guideline No. 70*, Edinburgh: SIGN.

Sikorski, J., Pindoria, S. and Wade, A. (2002) Support for Breastfeeding Mothers [Review], *Cochrane Database of Systematic Reviews*: Art. No.: 2002:CD001141.

Simmer, K., Patole, S. and Rao, S. (2008) Longchain Polyunsaturated Fatty Acid Supplementation in Infants Born at Term, *Cochrane Database of Systematic Reviews*, 1: Art. No. CD000376. DOI: 10.1002/14651858.CD000376.pub2.

Singhal, A. (2001) Early Nutrition in Preterm Infants and Later Blood Pressure: Two Cohorts after Randomised Trials, *Lancet*, 357: 413–19.

Smale, M., Renfrew, M., Marshall, J. *et al.* (2006) Turning Policy into Practice: More Difficult Than it Seems: The Case of Breastfeeding Education, *Maternal and Child Nutrition*, 2(2): 103–13.

Smith, A. (2002) Breast Pathology, in M. Walker (ed.) *Core Curriculum for Lactation Consultant Practice*, London: Jones and Bartlett.

Souto, G., Giugliani, E., Giugliani, C. *et al.* (2003) The Impact of Breast Reduction Surgery on Breastfeeding Performance, *Journal of Human Lactation*, 19(43): 43–9.

Spear, H. (2004) Nurses' Knowledge, Attitudes and Behaviours Related to the Promotion of Breastfeeding Among Women Who Bear Children During Adolescence, *Journal of Pediatric Nursing*, 19(3): 176–83.

Spencer, J. (2008) Management of Mastitis in Breastfeeding Women, *American Family Physician*, 78(6): 727–33.

Stables, D. and Rankin, J. (2010) *Physiology in Childbearing* (3rd edn), Edinburgh: Elsevier.

Sullivan-Boylai, J., Fife, K., Jacobs, R. *et al.* (2001) Disseminated Neonatal Herpes Simplex Virus Type 1 from a Maternal Breast Lesion, *Pediatrics*, 71(3): 456–8.

Tappin, D., Brown, A., Girdwood, R. *et al.* (2001) Breastfeeding Rates are Increasing in Scotland, *Health Bulletin*, 59(2): 102–7.

Tappin, D., Britten, J., Broadfoot, M. *et al.* (2006) The Effect of Health Visitors on Breastfeeding in Glasgow, *International Breastfeeding Journal*, 1(11). Available online at www.ncbi.nlm. nih.gov/pmc/articles/PMC1526418 (accessed 9 April 2011).

Taylor, J., Kacmar, J., Nothnagle, M. *et al.* (2005) A Systematic Review of the Literature Associating Breastfeeding with Type 2 Diabetes and Gestational Diabetes, *Journal of the American College of Nutrition*, 24(5): 320–6.

Tender, J., Janakiram, J. and Arce, J. (2009) Reasons for In-hospital Formula Supplementation of Breastfed Infants from Low Income Families, *Journal of Human Lactation*, 25: 11–17.

Thompson, J., Heal, L., Roberts, C. *et al.* (2010) Women's Breastfeeding Experiences Following a Significant Primary Postpartum Haemorrhage: A Multicentre Cohort Study, *International Breastfeeding Journal*, 5(5).

Trotter, S. (2010) Raising Awareness Amongst Parents of Treatments for Tongue-tie, *MIDIRS Midwifery Digest*, 20(1): 83–5.

UNICEF (n.d.) *Best Practice Standards for Establishing and Maintaining Lactation and Breastfeeding in Neonatal Units.* Available online at www.babyfriendly.org.uk/pdfs/neonatal_standards.pdf (accessed 8 April 2011).

UNICEF (1998) *Implementing the Ten Steps to Successful Breastfeeding*, London: UNICEF UK Baby Friendly Initiative.

UNICEF (2001) *Implementing the Baby Friendly Best Practice Standards: A Guide to Implementing the Ten Steps to Successful Breastfeeding and the Seven Point Plan for the Protection, Promotion and Support of Breastfeeding in Community Healthcare Settings*, London: UNICEF UK Baby Friendly Initiative.

UNICEF (2002) *Introducing the Baby Friendly Best Practice Standards into Breastfeeding Education for Student Midwives and Health Visitors*, London: UNICEF UK Baby Friendly Initiative.

UNICEF (2008a) *Three-day Course in Breastfeeding Management: Participants' Handbook*, London: UNICEF UK Baby Friendly Initiative.

UNICEF (2008b) *Guidance Notes for Implementing the Baby Friendly Initiative Education Standards: Higher Education Institutions*, London: UNICEF UK Baby Friendly Initiative.

UNICEF (2008c) *Best Practice Standards for Higher Education Institutions.* Available online at www.babyfriendly.org.uk/page.asp?page=129 (accessed 6 April 2011).

UNICEF (2009) *Guidance Notes for the Implementation of the Baby Friendly Initiative Standards: Higher Education Institutions.* Available online at www.babyfriendly.org.uk/pdfs/ed_stds_guidance.pdf (accessed 20 October 2009).

UNICEF (2010a) *The Baby Friendly Initiative: Baby Friendly Progress by Country.* Availbable online at http://www.babyfriendly.org.uk (accessed 5 September 2010).

UNICEF (2010b) *Baby Friendly Progress by Country.* Available online at www.babyfriendly.org.uk/htables/country_overview.asp (accessed 24 May 2010).

UNICEF (2010c) *Guidance on the Development of Policies and Guidelines for the Prevention and Management of Hypoglycaemia of the Newborn.* Available online at www.babyfriendly.org.uk (accessed 9 September 2010).

UNICEF (2010d) *The Health Professional's Guide To: 'A Guide to Infant Formula for Parents Who Are Bottle Feeding'*, London: UNICEF UK BFI.

UNICEF (2010e) *Hospital Initiative Review 2010*, London: UNICEF UK BFI.

van Veldhuizen-Staas, C. (2007) Overabundant Milk Supply: An Alternative Way to Intervene by Full Drainage and Block Feeding, *International Breastfeeding Journal*, 2(11). Available online at www.ncbi.nlm.nih.gov/pmc/articles/PMC2075483 (accessed 9 April 2011).

Vennemann, M., Bajanowski, T., Brinkmann, B. *et al.* (2009) Does Breastfeeding Reduce the Risk of Sudden Infant Death Syndrome? *Pediatrics*, 123(3): 406–10.

WABA (World Alliance for Breastfeeding Action) (2005) Towards Healthy Environments for Children: FAQs about Breastfeeding in a Contaminated Environment. Available online at www.waba.org.my/whatwedo/environment/pdf/faq2005_eng.pdf (accessed 9 April 2011).

WA Centre for Evidence Based Nursing & Midwifery (2007) *Breastfeeding Guidelines for Substance Abusing Mothers.* Available online at http://specosium.curtin.edu.au/breastfeeding/Infant%20Feeding_Guidelines.pdf (accessed 6 August 2010).

Walker, M. (2002) Maternal Breastfeeding Anatomy, in M. Walker (ed.) *Core Curriculum for Lactation Consultant Practice* (pp. 1–11), London: Jones and Bartlett Publishers.

Walker, M. (2010) *Breastfeeding Management and the Clinician: Using the Evidence*, London: Jones and Bartlett Publishers.

Walsh, M. and Wigens, L. (2003) *Introduction to Research*, Cheltenham: Nelson Thornes.

Watson-Genna, C. and Sandora, L. (2008) Breastfeeding: Normal Sucking and Swallowing, in C. Watson-Genna (ed.) *Supporting Sucking Skills in Breastfeeding Infants* (pp. 1–42), London: Jones and Bartlett Publishers.

White, J. (1995) Patterns of Knowing: Review, Critique, and Update, *Advances in Nursing Science*, 17(4): 73–86.

WHO (World Health Organization) (1977) *Hypoglycaemia of the Newborn: Review of the Literature*, Geneva: WHO.

WHO (World Health Organization) (1981) *International Code of Marketing of Breast Milk Substitutes*, Geneva: WHO.

WHO (World Health Organization) (1990) *Innocenti Declaration on the Protection, Promotion and Support of Breastfeeding*, Florence: WHO.

WHO (World Health Organization) (1998a) *Evidence for the Ten Steps to Successful Breastfeeding*, Geneva: WHO.

WHO (World Health Organization) (1998b) *Relactation: Review of Experience and Recommendations for Practice*, Geneva: WHO.

WHO (World Health Organization) (2002) *Infant and Young Child Nutrition: Global Strategy on Infant and Young Child Feeding*, Geneva: 55th World Health Assembly.

WHO (World Health Organization) (2003) *Managing Newborn Problems: A Guide for Doctors, Nurses and Midwives*, Geneva: WHO.

WHO (World Health Organization) (2010a) *10 Facts on Breastfeeding*. Available online at www.who.int/features/factfiles/breastfeeding/en (8 April 2011).

WHO (World Health Organization) (2010b) *Guidelines on HIV and Infant Feeding: Principles and Recommendations for Infant Feeding in the Context of HIV and a Summary of Evidence*, Geneva: WHO.

WHO (World Health Organization)/UNICEF (1989) *Ten Steps to Successful Breastfeeding*, Geneva: WHO. Available online at www.unicef.org/newsline/tensteps.htm (accessed 6 April 2011).

WHO (World Health Organization)/UNICEF (2009) *Acceptable Medical Reasons for the Use of Breast-milk Substitutes*, Geneva: WHO.

Wilde, C., Addey, C., Boddy, L. *et al.* (1995) Autocrine Regulation of Milk Secretion by a Protein in Milk, *Biochemistry Journal*, 1(305): 51–8.

Willis, C. and Livingstone, V. (1995) Infant Insufficient Milk Syndrome Associated with Maternal Postpartum Haemorrhage, *Journal of Human Lactation*, 11: 123–6.

Woolridge, M. and Drewett, R. (1986) Sucking Rates of Human Babies on the Breast: A Study using Direct Observation, *Journal of Reproductive and Infant Psychology*, 4(1–2): 69–75.

Woolridge, M., Baum, J. and Drewett, R. (1980) Effect of a Traditional and a New Nipple Shield on Sucking Patterns and Milk Flow, *Early Human Development*, 4(4): 357–64.

Worgan, R. (2002) Induced Lactation and Relactation, in M. Walker (ed.) *Core Curriculum for Lactation Consultant Practice* (pp. 230–46), London: Jones and Bartlett.

Index

Note: page references to boxes, figures or tables are in *italic* print.